100 Challenges in Echocardiography

For Elsevier:

Commissioning Editor: Alison Taylor
Development Editor: Kim Benson
Production Manager: Susan Stuart
Design and Production: Helius
Illustrations: Pierrick Cordonnier
Translation: Quarto Translations

100 Challenges in Echocardiography

CHRISTOPHE KLIMCZAK MD PhD

*Cardiologist and Hospital Practitioner, University Hospital Paris VI
(Pierre & Marie Curie): Charles Foix and Emile Roux;
Expert in Echocardiography, Cardiovascular Institute, Paris, France*

Consultant Editor for the English language edition:
Petros Nihoyannopoulos MD FRCP FACC FESC
*Consultant Cardiologist, Imperial College School of Medicine,
Hammersmith Hospital, London, UK; President, European Association
of Echocardiography of the ESC*

ELSEVIER

EDINBURGH • LONDON • NEW YORK • OXFORD • PHILADELPHIA
ST LOUIS • SYDNEY • TORONTO • 2008

ELSEVIER

100 pièges en échocardiographie, 1ère édition
© Elsevier Masson SAS, Paris, 2005

© 2008, this translation, Elsevier Limited. All rights reserved.
First published 2008

ISBN: 978-0-443-06927-7

British Library Cataloguing in Publication Data
A catalogue record for this book is available from the British Library.

Library of Congress Cataloging in Publication Data
A catalog record for this book is available from the Library of Congress.

Note

Knowledge and best practice in this field are constantly changing. As new research and experience broaden our knowledge, changes in practice, treatment and drug therapy may become necessary or appropriate. Readers are advised to check the most current information provided (i) on procedures featured or (ii) by the manufacturer of each product to be administered, to verify the recommended dose or formula, the method and duration of administration, and contraindications. It is the responsibility of the practitioner, relying on their own experience and knowledge of the patient, to make diagnoses, to determine dosages and the best treatment for each individual patient, and to take all appropriate safety precautions. To the fullest extent of the law, neither the Publisher nor the Author assumes any liability for any injury and/or damage to persons or property arising out or related to any use of the material contained in this book.   *The Publisher*

Printed in China

Contents

Acknowledgements

The author would like to thank the following people for their contribution to the illustrations in this book:

- Kontron Médical, an Esaote group company
- Doctor Dominique Guedj-Meynier, President of the National College of French Cardiologists
- Professor Raymond Roudaut of the Cardiology University Hospital Haut-Lévêque, Bordeaux, France
- Doctors Janusz Kochanowski and Piotr Scislo of the cardiology clinic of the Warsaw Academy of Medicine (Professor G. Opolski), Poland.

This book is dedicated in respectful homage to my compatriot Marie Curie-Sklodowska (1867–1934), who, through her scientific discovery of radioactivity, gave birth to nuclear medicine. The University of Paris VI has chosen her name as its emblem.

Christophe Klimczak

Abbreviations

2D	two-dimensional		HCM	hypertrophic cardiomyopathy
Aa	annular A wave		HOCM	hypertrphic obstructive cardiomyopathy
AC	anterior commissure		HR	heart rate
An	annulus		HVF	hepatic venous flow
AN	aneurysm			
AO	aorta		IAS	interatrial septum
AR	aortic regurgitation		IVC	interventricular communication
AS	aortic stenosis			
AT	acceleration time		IVRT	isovolumic relaxation time
ASE	American Society of Echocardiography		IVS	interventricular septum
AOC	aortic closing		IVST	interventricular septal thickness
AOO	aortic opening			
ASH	asymmetrical septal hypertrophy		LA	left atrium
			LAA	left atrial appendage
D	diameter		LAR	left auricle
DDT	D wave deceleration time		LCC	left coronary cusp
DT	deceleration time		LMV	large mitral valve
DTI	Doppler tissue imaging		LPV	left pulmonary vein
			LV	left ventricle
Co	coaptation		LVDA	left ventricular end-diastolic surface area
e	endocardium		LVH	left ventricular hypertrophy
Ea	annular E wave		LVM	left ventricular mass
ECG	electrocardiogram		LVSA	left ventricular end-systolic surface area
EDD	end-diastolic diameter			
EDP	end-diastolic pressure		MAd	mitral A wave duration
EDS	end-diastolic surface area		MC	mitral closing
EDT	E wave deceleration time		MF	mitral flow
EDV	end-diastolic volume		MI	myocardial infarction
EF	ejection fraction		MO	mitral opening
Em	mitral E wave		MR	mitral regurgitation
ESD	end-systolic diameter		MRI	magnetic resonance imaging
ESS	end-systolic surface area		MS	mitral stenosis
ESV	end-systolic volume		MSA	mitral surface area
Ex	endocardial excursion		MSC	midsystolic closure
Exp	paradoxical expansion			
FS	systolic fraction			

MVP	mitral valve prolapse		ROA	regurgitant orifice area
			RPV	right pulmonary vein
NCC	non-coronary cusp		RUPV	right upper pumonary vein
			RV	right ventricle
O_a	aortic output		RVEDP	right ventricular end-
O_m	mitral output			diastolic pressure
OCM	obstructive cardiomyopathy		RWT	relative wall thickness
OHCM	obstructive hypertrophic			
	cardiomyopathy		S	surface area
Pa	pulmonary artery		Sa	annular S wave
PA	amplitude of A wave		SAM	systolic anterior motion
PAd	duration of A wave of		SAOS	subaortic surface
	pulmonary venous flow		SAP	systolic arterial pressure
PAHT	pulmonary arterial		SF	shortening fraction
	hypertension		SHVF	subhepatic venous flow
PAP	pulmonary arterial pressure		SMV	small mitral valve
PAPd	diastolic pulmonary arterial		SSF	surface shortening fraction
	pressure			
PAPm	mean pulmonary arterial		$T_{\frac{1}{2}p}$	pressure half-time
	pressure		TC	tricuspid closing
PAPs	systolic pulmonary arterial		TEE	transoesophageal
	pressure			echocardiography
PAT	pulmonary arterial trunk		TGC	time gain compensation
PC	posterior commissure		Th	systolic thickening
PE	pericardial effusion		Tn	systolic thinning
PENN	Pennsylvania		TO	tricuspid opening
PET	pre-ejection time		TR	tricuspid regurgiation
PFM	pulse repetition frequency		Tric	tricuspid
PFO	patent foramen ovale		TTE	transthoracic
PHT	pressure half-time			echocardiography
PISA	proximal isovelocity surface			
	area		V	velocity
PLE	pleural effusion		V_1	velocity upstream of
PR	pulmonary regurgitation			stenosis
Pulm	pulmonary		V_2	velocity at the level of
Pv	propagation velocity			stenosis
PVF	pulmonary venous flow		V_{ed}	end-diastolic velocity
PW	posterior wall		V_{max}	maximum velocity
PWT	posterior wall thickness		V_{pd}	early diastolic velocity
			V_R	regurgitant volume
Q_{AO}	aortic output		VC	vena contracta
			VST	ventricular septal thickness
r	radius		VTI	velocity-time integral
RA	right atrium		VTI_{ao}	aortic velocity–time integral
RAP	right atrial pressure		VTI_{sao}	subaortic velocity–time
RCC	right coronary cusp			integral
RF	regurgitation fraction		VTRd	diastolic VTR
RO	regurgitated output		VTRs	systolic VTR

Forewords

For more than 15 years, Christophe Klimczak has been assisting cardiologists in their training through his many treatises on echocardiography (clinical, trans-oesophageal, stress, in elderly subjects). Through these publications, cardiologists have been able to appreciate the teaching and synthesis that characterize his writing.

This time, he has had the inspired notion of putting down on paper the 100 most common pitfalls in echocardiography – pitfalls which inexperienced echocardiographers, but also cardiologists, are likely to experience. The originality of this book resides primarily in its theme, which to my knowledge has never previously been discussed, but also in the exhaustiveness of its content, which encompasses both the physical principles of ultrasonic waves and current diagnoses in cardiology. The advantage of such an approach becomes clear when one is familiar with the potentially serious consequences of a wrongly interpreted echocardiograph, both in terms of the diagnosis, and of the prognosis and treatment.

Always closely in touch with clinical medicine and with patients, Christophe Klimczak has unquestionably achieved his goal of a collection that is both attractive and complete. This is a book that is destined to accompany the echocardiographer to the patient's bedside.

Professor Albert Hagège
Cardiology Department
Hôpital européen Georges Pompidou
Paris

Medical imaging in general, and echocardiography in particular, has seen considerable advances over the past two decades. The technological mastery of ultrasonic waves has made it possible to evolve from one-dimensional echocardiography to two- and three-dimensional echocardiography, from greyscale imaging to colour imaging, from external probes to external and internal probes, etc. The medical advances have allowed the evolution from the approximate evaluation of a single cardiac structure to a precise functional study of the myocardium, both in the basal state and during laboratory tests, such as under pharmacological or physical stress. This technical development has been accompanied by a broadening of the indications for echocardiography, leading to its widespread diffusion. Thus echocardiographers have abandoned their research centres and specialized units in order to form part of the daily examinations in private and hospital clinical laboratories.

The experience of the medical teams and the fantastic evolution of the equipment have contributed to defining with precision the indications for echocardiography and to establishing recommendations for its day-to-day use. As with other medical techniques, echocardiography should be carried out with numerous precautions and with certain rules observed in order to provide reliable and reproducible results. Thus, throughout the echocardiographic examination the cardiologist should proceed in a methodical manner in order to avoid the many potential pitfalls, the consequences of which would be regrettable. In short, there are pitfalls of echocardiography at each stage of the examination, both in recording and in interpretation; hence the need for a detailed focus on the subject.

My colleague and friend Dr Christophe Klimczak has dedicated a considerable part of his professional life to echocardiography. He is manager of several echocardiographic units and has enormous experience in this field. Dr Klimczak has carried out numerous scientific endeavours and is the author of several reference works on echocardiography. He is therefore particularly well positioned to share his experience and provide a focus, which is both comprehensive and pragmatic, on the pitfalls to be avoided in echocardiography.

The book Dr Klimczak has written is both didactic and rich in illustrations. The reader will appreciate the many tables, figures, examples and simulations of pitfalls, which clarify the exposition and confirm the author's pedagogical qualities. These elements will ensure that cardiologists, both private doctors and hospital practitioners, will undoubtedly appreciate the significant work that Dr Klimczak displays in this book.

Professor Roland Asmar
The Cardiovascular Institute
Clinique Mozart
Paris

Preface

There has been enormous progress in echocardiography over the past 30 years, and today it is considered probably the most important, first-line imaging modality for the heart. The unique advantage of the technique is the lack of radiation, which significantly limits the use of nuclear modalities. A further advantage is its ready availability worldwide, which brings it close to the patient. The biggest limitation of echocardiography, however, derives, paradoxically, from its advantages, but also from the lack of regulatory authorities to regulate the practice of echocardiography by those who are recognized experts or trained specialists. The European Association of Echocardiography has taken the unprecedented step of accrediting individuals and laboratories around Europe into the practice of echocardiography, which will raise European standards uniformly.

This book by Christophe Klimczak on the 100 challenges in echocardiography is unique, in that it focuses on the most frequent pitfalls and interpretation problems that one may encounter during a routine echocardiographic examination. This alone highlights the need for subspecialist training in echocardiography, and this book will certainly become a necessity for all those who start performing echocardiography, and in particular those who wish to become experts.

Petros Nihoyannopoulos
Professor of Cardiology
President, European Association
of Echocardiography of the ESC

Introduction

Echocardiography is a cardiac investigation based on the use of ultrasonic waves. It enables an anatomical and functional description of the heart. Carried out in the traditional manner by the transoesophageal route, echocardiography has become an irreplaceable routine instrument in day-to-day cardiological clinical practice. It provides information of a diagnostic, therapeutic and prognostic nature. For these reasons, echocardiographic examination should be carried out in a rigorous manner by a competent doctor specializing in echocardiography. A doctor who has had sufficient theoretical and practical training is the most suitable person to correctly carry out, and reliably interpret, the echocardiogram.

Echocardiography has today taken on the appearance of a multimodal technique (harmonic imaging, Doppler tissue imaging, transoesophageal exploration, three-dimensional reconstruction, etc.), and hence there is a need for a good knowledge of the limitations of this technique and of the numerous pitfalls that may be encountered during the course of such an examination.

These pitfalls may be:

- technical – principally due to the operator in relation to the examination
- diagnostic – in relation to the exploration of a specific cardiac anomaly.

Familiarity with these pitfalls will make it possible to avoid mistakes or incorrect interpretations of the examination, which can compromise the diagnosis or appropriate patient care. However, the echocardiographic data collected during the examination should always be put back into their clinical context and compared with other, complementary examinations.

The goal of this book is to discuss in a practical and didactic manner the pitfalls in echocardiography. The number '100' is symbolic, acknowledging the importance of the situations, sometimes complex and difficult to resolve, which the operator may face during the day-to-day practice of echocardiography. This work complements my series of books on echocardiography.

Christophe Klimczak

References

Klimczak C. *Échocardiographie Clinique.* Cardiologie Pratique. Masson, Paris, 2006.

Klimczak C. *Échographie Cardiaque Transoesophagienne.* Cardiologie Pratique. Masson, Paris, 2002.

Klimczak C. *Échographie Cardiaque de Stress.* Abrèges de Médecine. Masson, Paris, 1997.

SECTION I
Technical pitfalls

1

The physical limitations of echocardiography

The physical limitations of echocardiography are due to the physical properties of ultrasonic waves, the resolution of the echocardiogram and the aliasing phenomenon. Familiarity with these factors will make it easier to master the technique of diagnostic ultrasound.

PHYSICAL PROPERTIES OF ULTRASONIC WAVES

Ultrasonic waves emitted by piezoelectric crystals propagate at a constant speed in the myocardium and the blood (1540 m/s). By comparison, this propagation speed is far higher in bone (3380 m/s) and lower in air (354 m/s). As these two media are high absorbers of ultrasound, they are very poor conductors. Examinations are therefore often difficult in obese patients, or patients with emphysema, thoracic deformations or narrow intercostal spaces.

RESOLUTION OF AN ECHOCARDIOGRAM

The resolution of an echocardiogram, i.e. the capacity of the ultrasonic waves to distinguish between two anatomical structures that are spatially close to one another, or adjacent, varies directly with the emission frequencies of the ultrasonic waves and inversely with the wavelength of the ultrasound beam. With the frequencies habitually used in echocardiography (below 5 MHz), the so-called 'axial resolution' is in the range 0.6–1.6 mm. In practice, the lower the axial resolution, the better the detail of the image.

ALIASING PHENOMENON

The main disadvantage of pulsed Doppler echocardiography is the phenomenon of velocity ambiguity. In fact, the pulse repetition frequency (PRF) of the echocardiogram may be too low to measure high blood flow velocity (above 1–1.5 m/s). This situation gives rise to the phenomenon of aliasing, or spectral folding: the highest velocities are cut off the top of the spectrum and appear as a mirror image in the other direction (Fig. 1.1). In colour Doppler, which is a modality of pulsed Doppler, the aliasing phenomenon occurs for velocities above 0.8–1 m/s, in the form of a colour inversion. Familiarity with the aliasing phenomenon is vital in order to interpret correctly the Doppler data obtained.

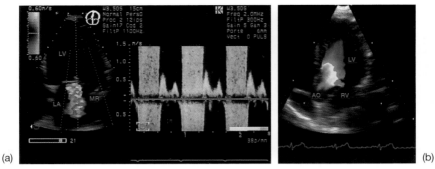

Figure 1.1 Aliasing phenomena in Doppler echocardiography: (a) pulsed mode (folded spectrum of mitral regurgitation); (b) two-dimensional colour mode (normal aortic ejection flow aliased in its maximum acceleration zone). AO, aorta; LA, left atrium; LV, left ventricle; MR, mitral regurgitation; RV, right ventricle.

2

Ultrasound artefacts

Echocardiography does not depart from the rules of medical imaging. As in radiography, the ultrasound image may contain a certain number of virtual images, called artefacts, that have no basis in reality. These false images, wrongly interpreted, may become diagnostic pitfalls for the clinician.

Ultrasound artefacts may be linked to:

- the physical limitations of the equipment used (e.g. limitations in resolution)
- an incorrect adjustment of the machine settings, particularly of the gain settings, when recording the image
- the anatomical structures themselves
- the patients themselves.

The first two potential sources of artefacts are correctable and are discussed further in Chapter 1. This leaves those artefacts that arise from transthoracic examinations (Figs 2.1 and 2.2):

- ultrasound reverberations
- the shadow cone
- posterior acoustic enhancement
- the black hole.

ULTRASOUND REVERBERATIONS

Ultrasound reverberation is the result of a ping-pong effect between the probe and a highly reflective medium such as air. On the basis of a single ultrasound emission, the instrument does not record a single return echo, but a burst of echoes. Only the first echo corresponds to the real image of the probe/air interface (first echogenic line). The echoes that follow are artefacts (reverberations) and form a succession of echogenic, arc-shaped lines, one behind the other, equidistant from the transducer. Such an image is obtained, for example, when there is an insufficient amount of gel between the probe and the skin, or simply when the probe is placed directly over a rib (rib effect). Adding more gel, or moving the probe slightly, will correct this artefact. The reverberations may also arise from other structures that produce echoes (hyperechoic structures) within the heart or the thorax. By readjusting the probe angle, these artefacts can sometimes be eliminated. So-called linear or mirror image artefacts concerning the thoracic aorta are discussed further on page 208.

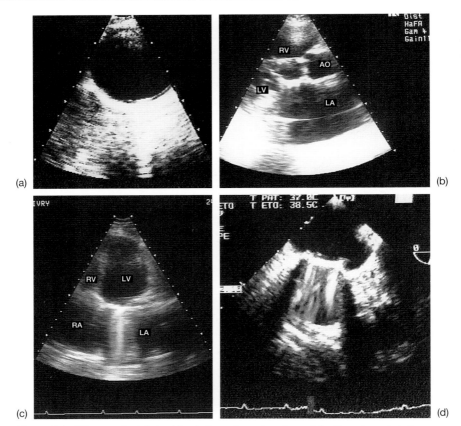

Figure 2.1   Ultrasound artefacts: (a) anterior wall reverberations of the thoracic aorta in trans-oesophageal echocardiography (TEE); (b) linear echo in the ectatic left atrium in transthoracic echocardiography (TTE); (c, d) shadow cone in a St. Jude mitral prosthesis in TTE (c) and in TEE (d). AO, aorta; LA, left atrium; LV, left ventricle; RA, right atrium; RV, right ventricle.

SHADOW CONE

The shadow cone corresponds to a loss of information behind a bone, calcified tissue or prosthetic material, due to a complete reflection of the ultrasound beam off these structures. It is an acoustic shadow that appears on the screen as a grey, sparkling area.

POSTERIOR ACOUSTIC ENHANCEMENT

Posterior acoustic enhancement is the formation of an image downstream of liquid structures (blood contained within the cardiac chambers), which attenuate the ultrasound only a little. This enhancement, which is manifested as a hyperenhancement of the tissues, may mask, for example, a small pericardial

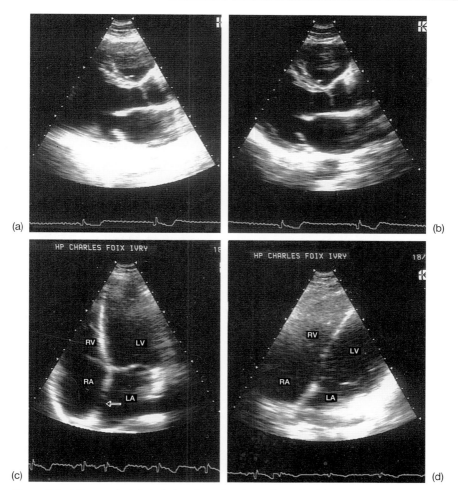

Figure 2.2 Ultrasound artefacts in transthoracic echocardiography: (a) posterior acoustic enhancement of the posterior wall of the left ventricle (LV), and (b) corrected by adjusting the gain; (c) black hole at the level of the interatrial septum (IAS) simulating an interatrial communication in an apical cross-section of the four chambers, but not visible in a subcostal cross-section (d) – continuity of the IAS is retained. LA, left atrium; LV, left ventricle; RA, right atrium; RV, right ventricle.

effusion. However, this artefact is easily corrected by reducing the gain towards the posterior wall.

BLACK HOLE

This artefact is most commonly an image of a virtual 'black hole' in the middle of the interatrial septum, and occurs when the ultrasound beam arrives parallel to the septum and does not produce any return echo (anechoic zone). Such an image can therefore lead to an incorrect diagnosis of interatrial communication. This error may be avoided by increasing the number of ultrasound projections, which allows the septum to be explored from different angles.

SUMMARY

In short, artefactual images may prove troublesome if they are not understood. They may also give rise to false interpretations of the echocardiogram. However, with the ongoing improvements in ultrasound techniques, these deceptive artefacts are becoming increasingly rare.

3
Patient hypoechogenicity

A patient's echogenicity is attributed to the 'acoustic impedance' phenomenon, which corresponds to the resistance offered by a particular tissue to the propagation of the ultrasound beam. Each constituent tissue of the thoracic cavity (skin, bone, lung, myocardium, etc.) possesses a different acoustic impedance. Two adjoining media of different impedances form an 'acoustic interface', which is capable of reflecting ultrasound beams. The greater the difference in impe-

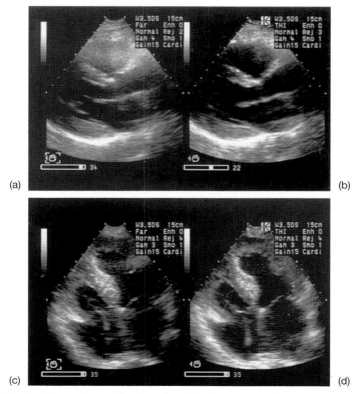

(a)   (b)

(c)   (d)

Figure 3.1   (a, c) Hypoechogenicity of a patient in fundamental two-dimensional imaging. (b, d) There is a clear improvement in image quality in the harmonic mode (better definition of the endocardium).

dance between the two media, the greater the reflection. A clear image of the interface is then obtained. The hypoechogenicity of certain patients is attributed to a relatively lower capacity of a tissue to reflect ultrasound. The reason for this phenomenon is still unknown. However, progress in ultrasound technology, such as the application of harmonic imaging, has made it possible to reduce considerably the number of poorly echoic patients (Fig. 3.1). This does not preclude those rare, completely anechoic patients, in whom echocardiographic examination is 'impossible'.

4

Problems due to adjustments of the machine settings

To a large extent the quality of an echocardiogram depends on the intrinsic parameters of the probe, but the clinician can still make use of a certain number of adjustments to the echocardiographic apparatus in order to improve the quality of a recording. However, these more or less numerous adjustments vary from one echocardiographic recording to the next. Echocardiography therefore remains an operator-dependent examination. The technical pitfalls resulting from the use of echocardiography concern echocardiographic imaging and Doppler echocardiography, as well as spectral Doppler (pulsed and continuous) and colour Doppler (Box 4.1).

Box 4.1   Pitfalls due to adjustments of the machine settings

Pitfalls of echocardiographic imaging
- Inappropriate selection of emission frequency
- Incorrect adjustment of the angle of the two-dimensional sector, reception gains, greyscale, reject, focus, etc.

Pitfalls of spectral Doppler
- Inappropriate selection of the emission frequency
- Incorrect adjustment of the reception gain, filter, sample volume, spectrum speed, etc.

Pitfalls of colour Doppler
- Inappropriate selection of the angle of the coloured sector or the colour range
- Imprecise adjustment of the colour gain

PITFALLS OF ECHOCARDIOGRAPHIC IMAGING (Fig. 4.1)

Inappropriate choice of emission frequency

It is vital to select the optimal emission frequency for the probe generating the ultrasonic waves according to the patient being examined and the diagnostic problem at hand. In general, this frequency falls in the range 2–3.5 MHz in adults and 4–7 MHz in children. A technology known as multifrequency echocardiography, based on the application of variable-frequency ultrasound probes (probes with large bandwidth), enables the operator to select a suitable frequency band for each patient. In fact, the emission frequency chosen is directly responsible for the quality of the image obtained. It is important to remember that the higher the frequency, the better the image resolution. However, at high frequencies the

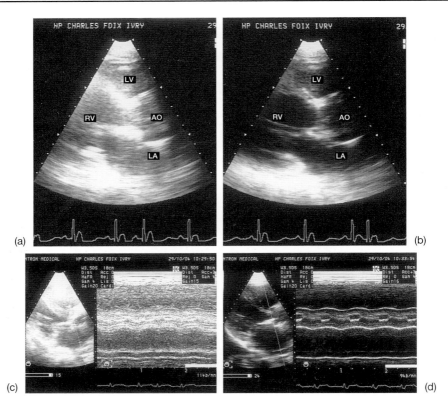

Figure 4.1   Pitfalls of imaging. Incorrect adjustment of the parameters in two-dimensional (a) and M-mode echocardiography masking the aortic opening (c). Correction of the adjustment, enabling perfect visualization of the cardiac structures (b, d). AO, aorta; LA, left atrium; LV, left ventricle; RV, right ventricle.

penetration energy of the ultrasonic waves is reduced. This results in an attenuation of the distal echoes, as the deep structures cannot be imaged.

In practice, the higher the emission frequency, the lower the exploration depth. What is required, therefore, is a compromise between frequency and exploration depth. The increasingly common use of what is known as 'harmonic imaging' makes it possible to improve further the quality of the echocardiographic image, and to obtain a better definition of the ventricular endocardium.

Incorrect adjustment of the angle of the sector field and the exploration depth

This adjustment depends, above all, on the volume of the heart to be analysed, the angle of the sector field (30–110°) and the exploration depth (2–23 cm). In general, the smaller the angle of exploration, the better the image resolution. However, in children the depth scale must be enlarged to avoid reverberations and to achieve optimal visualization of the structures to be studied. An adjustment button labelled 'angle' is available on some ultrasound machines; this enables the operator to vary the lateral position of the two-dimensional sector without modifying the position of the probe. This system makes possible a more profitable sectoral sweep of the cardiac structures.

Insufficient adjustment of the gains

Adjusting the gain controls makes it possible to adapt the reception level of the ultrasound signal without changing the intensity of the ultrasonic waves emitted. Such an adjustment is useful for limiting the phenomenon of attenuation of deep echoes. This attenuation is due to the absorption of the ultrasound beam by the tissues during exploration of the cardiac structures. Roughly speaking, the so-called 'total gain' is responsible for the general brightness of the image. There is often a tendency to work with an image that is too bright, as the eye is invariably attracted to this type of image. However, the saturation is such that the image may actually be 'burned', which makes it impossible to capture the details.

Due to attenuation of the beam by the tissue the echoes returning from deep structures are weaker than those from proximal structures. In order to compensate for this limitation, adjusting the gain for each depth level using sliding potentials (time gain compensation (TGC) system) allows the brightness of the echoes to be strengthened or reduced 1 cm of the exploration at a time. With the TGC system, a separate adjustment of the proximal or distal field makes it possible to locally reduce the superficial echoes that often saturate the image, and to strengthen deep echoes that are too attenuated, thereby avoiding loss of information.

Inappropriate selection of the greyscale

Appropriate selection of the greyscale (compression curve) enables an optimal distribution of the grey tones within the scale according to the ranges wherein the tissue information is situated.

An alternative system for colouring the image, with a choice of several palettes, can be used in order better to visualize certain echo structures, such as the myocardial walls in movement. This evaluation, however, appears to be somewhat subjective.

Incorrect adjustment of the dynamic echo scale

The dynamic echo scale (reject) makes it possible to increase the contrast by reducing the weaker echoes and intensifying the stronger echoes. It is the equivalent of a filter, enabling the partial elimination of ultrasound chatter in the reception. However, it should not be used at too high a level, as this would suppress useful echocardiographic signals.

Failure to use the focalization system

The focalization system makes it possible to converge the ultrasound beam onto one or more points (focal zones) of the image. It therefore enables an improvement of the resolution, and thus the image quality, in one or more precise zones that are of particular interest to the clinician.

PITFALLS OF SPECTRAL DOPPLER (Fig. 4.2)

Inappropriate selection of the emission frequency of the ultrasonic waves

This Doppler frequency, which can be adjusted by the user, varies according to the recording mode: pulsed or continuous Doppler. Continuous Doppler requires the use of the low frequency probe (preferably 2 MHz), making it possible to measure high blood flow velocities without limitation.

Incorrect adjustment of the reception gain of the spectrum

Incorrect adjustment of this control can skew the information about the velocity of the intracardiac flows under study.

Inappropriate adjustment of the rejection filter

The rejection filter enables the elimination of noise arising from the walls during slow movement of the valves. In practice, the rejection filter is usually adjusted to 200–400 Hz in pulsed Doppler and 800–1200 Hz in continuous Doppler. The result is better spectrum quality (intensity and clarity).

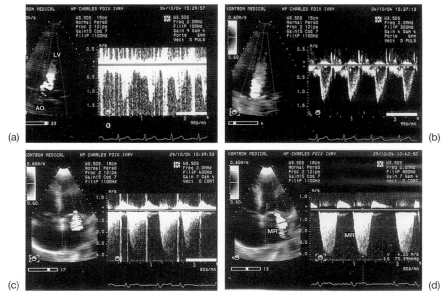

Figure 4.2 Pitfalls of spectral Doppler. (a, c) Incorrect adjustment of the gains and filters. Correction of the Doppler parameters enables clear visualization of (b) the contours of the 'interior void' spectrum of the aortic flow in pulsed mode and (d) of the 'full' spectrum of the mitral regurgitation (MR) jet in continuous mode. AO, aorta; LV, left ventricle.

Inappropriate selection of the sampling volume in pulsed Doppler

Appropriate selection of the sampling volume (Doppler gate 2–20 mm) makes it possible to improve the sensitivity and the resolution of the Doppler signal. The most commonly used average value of the Doppler gate (sample volume) is of the order of 4–6 mm.

Suboptimal adjustment of the spectrum speed

Echocardiographic traces can be collected at various speeds, the most commonly used being between 20 and 50 mm/s. In the case of rapid event analysis, it is possible to adjust the speed to 75 or 100 mm/s. This adjustment makes it possible to improve the precision of the Doppler measurements and to interpret correctly the data collected. It is vital to analyse the spectral curve simultaneously with an electrocardiographic trace, which provides a time reference for the cardiac cycle.

PITFALLS OF COLOUR DOPPLER (Fig. 4.3)

Imprecise adjustment of the general colour gain

This gain controls the reception of the Doppler signal. The adjustment is used to optimize the visualization of colour-coded intracardiac flows.

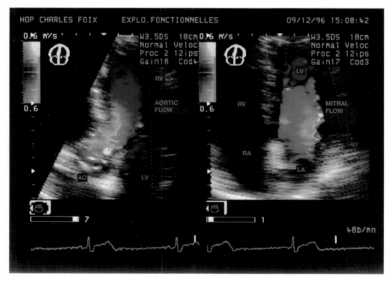

(a)   (b)

Figure 4.3 Correct recording of the normal flows in two-dimensional colour Doppler by the apical route (images in zoom): (a) aortic flow; (b) mitral flow. AO, aorta; LA, left atrium; LV, left ventricle; RA, right atrium; RV, right ventricle.

Unsuitable choice of angle of the two-dimensional coloured sector

The smallest angle of the two-dimensional coloured sector corresponds to the widest sweep frequency, which increases the sensitivity of the Doppler signal received.

Inappropriate choice of colour range

The choice of colour 'palette' is a function of the medical application of colour Doppler (cardiac or vascular exploration). It makes it possible preferentially to identify either low or high blood flow speeds. The choice of palette is also subjective, according to what an operator is accustomed to, and to his or her visual perception of colours on the screen. The visualization of turbulence (coded green) is optional and depends on the diagnostic question at hand.

5

Other technical pitfalls

Other technical pitfalls (Fig. 5.1) arise when the examination is uncomfortable for the operator because of:

- A technically difficult direction of approach, preventing the operator from locating an 'acoustic window' (i.e. a zone of exploration of the heart where the penetration of the ultrasonic waves is optimal) with the probe.
- A physical inability of the patient to assume certain positions (e.g. lying on their side) for the examination (e.g. an elderly patient, an incapacitating neurological or rheumatological condition, lack of cooperation from a child, intubated and ventilated patients).
- Particular situations that impede the passage of ultrasonic waves (e.g. a hairy torso, so that there is no firm probe–skin contact; large breasts; postoperative scars; thoracic dressing; drains; mammary prosthesis; artificial ventilation).

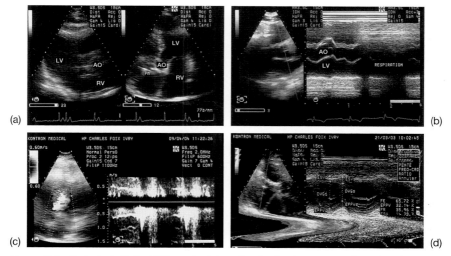

Figure 5.1 Technical pitfalls. (a) Thoracic deformation leading to poor two-dimensional image quality in the parasternal cross-section, which is compensated for by a good view in the apical cross-section. (b) Excessive respiration impeding the recording of the echocardiogram. (c) Technical breakdown of the continuous Doppler mode, creating noise in the spectrum. (d) Breakdown of the printer, deforming the echocardiographic trace. AO, aorta; LV, left ventricle; RV, right ventricle.

- Excessive respiratory movements, which can impede the acquisition of images when moving the probe closer to and further away from the cardiac structures. Moreover, the pulmonary lobes may become interposed between the probe and the heart. It is therefore sometimes necessary to ask patients to empty their lungs and to hold their breath for a few moments in order to achieve immobility of the thorax, and enable clear image capture.
- A fault in the distribution of the echocardiographic gel on the patient's skin, leading to a poor air–skin interface.

In summary, even if the echocardiographic examination is not of good technical quality in such situations, the information obtained can be used to resolve some simple problems. This is where the operator's experience and skill come into play.

SECTION II
Diagnostic pitfalls

6

Cardiac valves

VALVULAR STENOSES

Echocardiographic diagnosis of valvular stenoses, such as mitral stenosis (MS) or aortic stenosis (AS), is based on the study of:

- the morphology and motion of the stenotic valve
- the degree of valvular stenosis
- the haemodynamic consequences of the valvular stenosis.

PITFALLS WHEN STUDYING THE CONDITION OF THE STENOTIC VALVE

These echocardiographic pitfalls comprise:

- incomplete visualization of the stenotic valve
- imprecise assessment of the valvular lesions (morphology, mobility)
- particular cases, such as subvalvular MS or a bicuspid aortic valve.

Incomplete visualization of the valves (Fig. 6.1)

In order to assess correctly the condition of the stenotic valve, it is necessary to visualize:

- all the segments of the large and the small mitral valve (Fig. 6.2)
- the three semiluminal cusps of the aortic valve (Fig. 6.3)
- the valve commissures
- the chordae and papillary muscles of the mitral valve.

It may be necessary to resort to transoesophageal echocardiography (TEE), especially in the case of MS.

Imprecise evaluation of the degree of valvular and/or subvalvular remodelling (Fig. 6.4)

It may be difficult to evaluate the degree of valvular and/or subvalvular remodelling (fibrosis, calcification, commissural fusion, subvalvular retraction, etc.) due to:

- a possible non-uniformity of the valve lesion(s)
- a failure to use multiple projections
- an incorrect adjustment, particularly of the gain settings, which may lead to an over- or underestimation of the severity of stenosis.

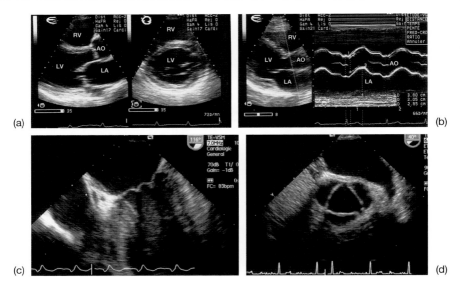

(a)   (b)

(c)   (d)

Figure 6.1   Normal valve appearance. Mitral valve viewed in (a) the longitudinal and transverse parasternal transthoracic echocardiography (TTE) cross-section and (c) in the multiplanar transoesophageal echocardiography (TEE) mode identifying the three mitral segments. Aortic valve viewed in (b) TTE (two-dimensional (2D)/M-mode) and (d) in the transverse TEE view showing the three open scallops and the commissures. AO, aorta; LA, left atrium; LV, left ventricle; RV, right ventricle.

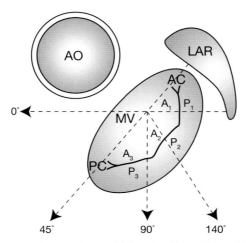

Figure 6.2   Segmentation of the mitral valve (MV) explored in multiplanar TEE: three segments of the large mitral valve (A_1, A_2, A_3) and three segments of the small mitral valve (P_1, P_2, P_3). The two mitral valve leaflets are separated by two commissures: the anterior commissure (AC) between A_1 and P_1, and the posterior commissure (PC) between A_3 and P_3. The TEE planes that can be used to study the different mitral segments are: 0°, A_1 and P_1; 45°, AC and PC; 90°, A_3 and P_3; 140°, A_2 and P_2. AO, aorta; LAR, left auricle.

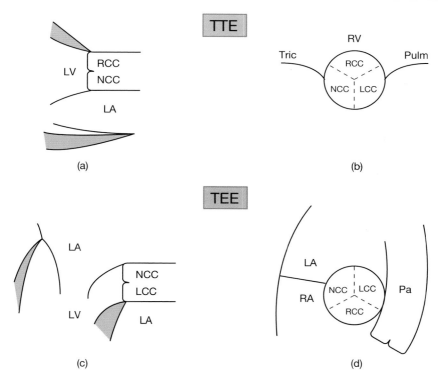

Figure 6.3   Two-dimensional cross-sections centred on the aortic orifice: (a) longitudinal and (b) transverse, parasternal TTE cross-sections; (c) major axis, multiplanar (110–130°) TEE cross-section; (d) minor axis multiplanar (60–80°) TEE cross-section. LA, left atrium; LCC, left coronary cusp; LV, left ventricle; NCC, non-coronary cusp; Pa, pulmonary artery; Pulm, pulmonary valve; RA, right atrium; RCC, right coronary cusp; RV, right ventricle; Tric, tricuspid valve.

The differential diagnosis between calcifications and fibrous nodules is not always simple. Generally, calcifications are manifested as dense and bright echoes that persist after reducing the gain settings. They are definite in the presence of an adjacent shadow cone. However, they are nonetheless quite frequently overestimated in echocardiograms.

Particular cases

Difficulty in appreciating valve mobility in the case of major calcification of the valves

It is often difficult to appreciate valve mobility when there is major calcification of the valves, which become hyperechoic and reverberating.

Failure to identify subvalvular mitral stenosis

This difficulty is due to the fusion and/or retraction of the chordae as well as fibrosis of the papillary muscles responsible for a subvalvular MS. In fact, the

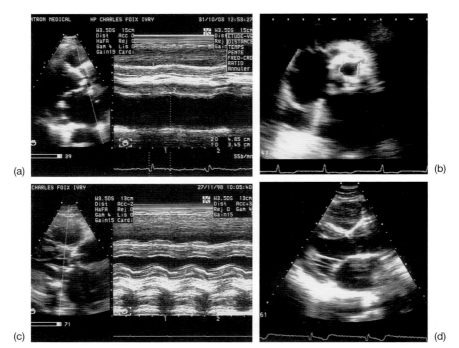

Figure 6.4   Valvular stenoses in TTE. (a) Calcifications of the aortic cusps masking the systolic opening in M-mode TTE. (b) Calcified and stenotic aortic orifice, evaluated at 1.02 cm² using planimetry. (c) Massive calcifications of the mitral annulus limiting valvular mobility. (d) Thickening and retraction of the mitral chordae in a case of mitral stenosis.

study of the subvalvular apparatus is more difficult than that of the valves, probably because subvalvular lesions are more complex and are often not easily picked up by transthoracic echocardiography (TTE). Identification of such lesions is much more precise in TEE.

Failure to diagnose a bicuspid aortic valve

It is sometimes difficult to identify a bicuspid valve when using TTE, as the extent of calcification does not allow for good definition of the commissures or the number of semilunar cusps. TEE is useful in this diagnosis. A quadricuspid aortic valve is a rare cardiac anomaly, and is generally responsible for AS.

Three-dimensional echocardiography appears to be advantageous in the study of the morphology and motion of stenotic cardiac valves (Fig. 6.5).

PITFALLS WHEN STUDYING THE DEGREE OF VALVULAR STENOSIS

The echocardiographic measurements that enable the quantification of valvular stenosis are:

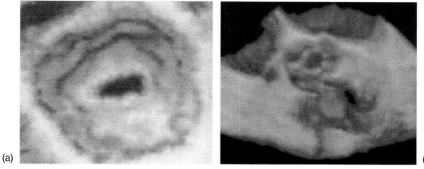

(a)   (b)

Figure 6.5 Three-dimensional reconstruction of (a) MS and (b) AS. (Images by Dr N. Mirochnik.)

- the trans-stenotic pressure gradient measured using continuous Doppler
- the surface area of the stenotic orifice:
  - anatomical (independent of the cardiac output), assessed using planimetry
  - functional (depending on the cardiac output), measured using Hatle's method (MS), the continuity equation (MS and AS) or the proximal isovelocity surface area (PISA) method (MS).

Each echo Doppler method has preferential indications and its own limitations. The elements that distinguish between the aortic surface area measured using echocardiography and that calculated using echo Doppler are summarized in Table 6.1.

Pitfalls when measuring the trans-stenotic pressure gradient (Box 6.1)

Absence of mean pressure gradient measurement
The mean pressure gradient better reflects the severity of the valvular stenosis than does the maximuml gradient. The mean value represents the integration

Table 6.1 Parameters that differ between the aortic surface area measured using echocardiography and that calculated using Doppler

	Echocardiographic surface area	Doppler surface area
Type of surface	Anatomical	Functional
Measurement mode	Planimetry	Continuity equation
Measurement site	Upstream of the vena contracta	At the level of the vena contracta
Relation to cardiac output	Independent of output	Dependent on output
Modification under Dobutamine	Fixed	Increased

> **Box 6.1   Pitfalls when measuring the trans-stenotic gradient using echo Doppler**
>
> - Failure to measure the mean gradient
> - Incomplete recording of stenotic jet
> - Failure to interpret the gradient as a function of the output and the cardiac frequency
> - Particular cases:
>   - inappropriate use of Bernoulli's equation
>   - neglect of the phenomenon of restoration of pressure

of the instantaneous gradient over the entire duration of the diastole (MS) or systole (AS). To calculate the mean gradient requires the maximum velocities in the central and proximal parts of the stenotic jet must be recorded. These measurements can be done using TEE, but TTE is generally adequate.

Incomplete recording of the stenotic jet when using continuous Doppler

Incomplete recording of the stenotic jet when using continuous Doppler can arise due to:

- technical impossibility, i.e. absence of the valid echocardiographic projection
- imperfect alignment of the Doppler beam with the stenotic jet (risk of under-estimating the gradient)
- failure to use different projections in order to obtain the highest possible velocities (in practice all echocardiographic projections should be used, bearing in mind that the apical windows (MS and AS) and right parasternal (AS) windows are the most 'profitable')
- incorrect adjustment, particularly of the gain and filter settings that determine the quality of the Doppler spectrum (the operator should make every effort to obtain a laminar flow with a well-defined spectral envelope, making use of colour Doppler and Doppler ultrasound).

Failure to interpret the stenotic gradient according to the blood output through the stenotic orifice and the heart rate

The severity of stenosis may be overestimated (increased gradient) due to a high cardiac output (anaemia, hyperthyroidism) or an associated valvular leak, or may be underestimated (reduced gradient) due to a low cardiac output linked to a systolic dysfunction of the left ventricle (LV). For example, a moderate mean gradient does not allow a tight valvular stenosis to be ruled out in a case of low cardiac output. Finally, for patients in atrial fibrillation, the averaging of several cycles is vital, taking into account the wide variability of the gradient according to the length of the cycles (Fig. 6.6).

Inappropriate use of the simplified Bernoulli equation in calculating the transvalvular gradient

The simplified Bernoulli equation ($4V_2^2$) is only valid if the velocity upstream of the stenosis (V_1) is insignificant compared with the velocity at the level of

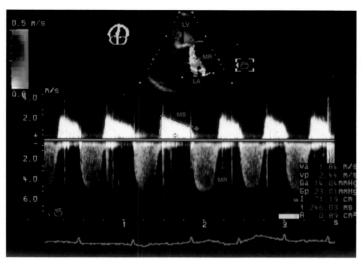

Figure 6.6 Mitral condition. Recording in continuous Doppler coupled with 2D colour imaging. The stenotic gradient and pressure half-time (PHT) (and therefore the mitral surface area (MSA)) vary due to the continuous arrhythmia arising from atrial fibrillation. LA, left atrium; LV, left ventricle; MR, mitral regurgitation; MS, mitral stenosis.

the stenosis (V_2). Otherwise (e.g. when the subaortic velocity is above 1.5 m/s) the use of the simplified equation leads to an overestimation of the gradient. The 'complete' Bernoulli formula $4(V_2{}^2 - V_1{}^2)$ should be used in this case.

Neglect of the phenomenon of restoration of pressure in the case of aortic stenosis

In general, this phenomenon is due to the difference in gradient between the vena contracta (Doppler), on the one hand, and the prestenotic zone and post-stenotic zone (catheterization) on the other. It equates to a retransformation, downstream of the vena contracta (zone of lowest pressure and highest velocity), of the kinetic energy into potential energy (remounting of pressure). This phenomenon leads to an overestimation of the gradients when using Doppler compared with those measured using catheterization. It can be observed in particular cases:

- in an adult, AS with an ascending aorta of small calibre (diameter < 30 mm)
- hourglass stenoses of the aortic coarctation type
- AS with high output.

Pitfalls when maesuring the surface area of the stenotic orifice

Pitfalls when using planimetry (Box 6.2)
Planimetry of the stenotic aortic orifice
Planimetry of the aortic orifice using two-dimensional (2D) TTE and the fundamental imaging method is practically impossible (small, irregular, ill-defined

---

> **Box 6.2   Pitfalls of planimetry of the mitral orifice**
>
> - Low echogenicity of the patient examined
> - Recording errors in the:
>   - adjustment of the gain settings
>   - choice of planimetry site
>   - tracking of the early diastole
> - Particular forms of the stenotic valve (membrane, funnel)
> - Major calcifications of the mitral orifice
> - Subvalvular mitral obstacle
> - In the case of atrial fibrillation
> - After balloon mitral valvuloplasty

orifice, hyperechoic valves). Harmonic imaging can be useful in better identifying the limits of the orifice (see Fig. 6.4(b)). Multiplanar TEE can be used to measure the aortic orifice by planimetry with good reliability. However, this method should be reserved for cases where the continuity equation cannot be used or where there is a discrepancy between the results obtained with different quantification methods.

Planimetry of the stenotic mitral orifice

Planimetry of the stenotic mitral orifice remains the most reliable method for determining what is known as the anatomical mitral surface area (MSA). It is carried out on the valve in the open position according to the transverse, parasternal, transthoracic cross-section, using the zoom and the cine loop function. This planimetric technique must be undertaken with particular care, as there are numerous possible pitfalls with this measurement, such as:

- Low echogenicity of the patient will prevent the operator from obtaining an adequate image of the mitral orifice (this is the cause of failure of the method in around 10% of cases).
- Recording errors in:
  - The adjustment of the gain settings, leading to a false definition of the internal limits of the mitral orifice: too low a gain leads to a falsely enlarged mitral orifice; too high a gain leads to a false image of an overly stenotic orifice.
  - The choice of planimetry site, either upstream of the free extremity of the mitral valve or, according to the 2D plane, oblique to the mitral orifice. These inappropriate views (Fig. 6.7) lead to an overestimation of the actual MSA (Fig. 6.8). In order to obtain a true value of the MSA, the operator must repeat the sweeps of the aorta towards the point of the LV in order to locate the mitral orifice. The cross-sectional plane must be perpendicular to the extremity of the mitral valves. Several planimetric measurements should be made and the mean value retained.

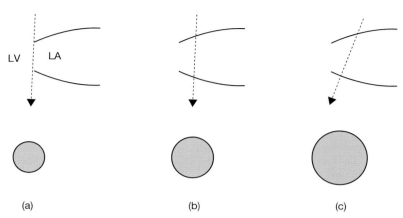

LV   LA

(a)   (b)   (c)

Figure 6.7   Mitral planimetry sites. (a) Correct site giving the actual MSA. Sites underestimating the MSA: (b) intravalvular; (c) oblique transvalvular. LA, left atrium; LV, left ventricle.

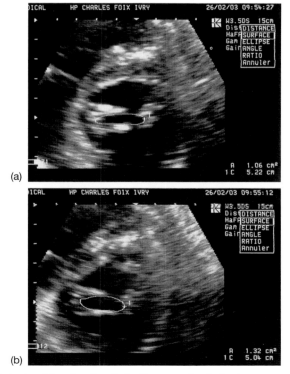

(a)

(b)

Figure 6.8   Planimetry of the stenotic mitral orifice according to the transverse, parasternal cross-section (zoomed 2D images). The mitral surface area (a) correctly measured using planimetry (1.06 cm²) and (b) overestimated (1.32 cm²) due to using the oblique 2D projection of the mitral orifice in the same patient.

- The tracking of the early diastole, which corresponds to the maximum opening of the mitral valve. Mid-diastolic planimetry leads to an under-estimation of the actual MSA.
- The particular morphological form of the stenotic valve (Fig. 6.9). An inappro-priate 2D cross-section of a very thin valve (known as non-calcified (soft-valve) MS) may incorrectly overestimate the area when compared with the rigid-valve (calcified valve) MS in the form of a funnel (Fig. 6.10).
- The presence of major calcifications of the mitral orifice, the reflected echoes of which can lead to an underestimation of the actual MSA.
- The presence of major remodelling of the subvalvular mitral apparatus (Fig. 6.11). The possibility of a predominantly subvalvular obstacle should be considered when the surface area measured using planimetry is greater than that calculated using Hatle's method (see below).
- Cases of atrial fibrillation. In order to obtain a precise value of the MSA, it is necessary to slow down the cardiac frequency.
- Following percutaneous mitral valve disease, measurement errors are poss-ible when using planimetry due to neglect of the scarcely visible limit of the open commissures and of the distorted form of the mitral orifice.

It should be noted that mitral planimetry is valuable in cases of associated mitral regurgitation (MR) or aortic regurgitation (AR).

Pitfalls when using Hatle's method

Hatle's method can be used to calculate the 'functional MSA' on the basis of the diastolic mitral flow recorded using continuous Doppler. This MSA value is based on the measurement of the pressure half-time (PHT), which varies in inverse proportion to the anatomical surface area of the mitral orifice. The MSA is derived from an empirical mathematical equation:

$$\text{MSA (cm}^2) = 220/\text{PHT (ms)}$$

This method may be used with TTE or TEE, but the transthoracic approach is generally sufficient.

Hatle's method is useful because it gives information about both valvular obstructions (commissural fusion) and subvalvular obstructions (lesions of the subvalvular apparatus), whereas planimetry gives information only about valvu-lar obstructions. When the PHT is carefully measured, the reliability of Hatle's method is excellent. Nevertheless, this method is not without several pitfalls (Box 6.3), which are described below.

Imperfect definition of the spectral envelope of the diastolic mitral flow

Imperfect definition of the spectral envelope of the diastolic mitral flow hinders the determination of the deceleration slope. Such poor definition arises due to:

- non-alignment with the stenotic jet
- incorrect adjustment of the gain or filter settings
- associated AR, leading to fluttering of the mitral slope.

Obtaining an interpretable Doppler curve with unambiguously defined contours is of primary importance.

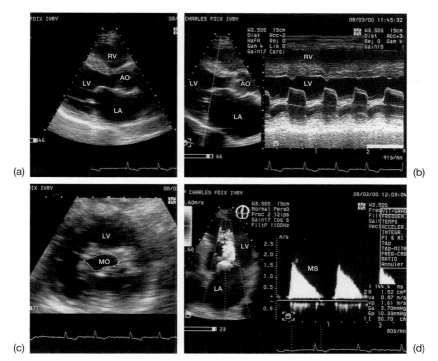

Figure 6.9   Slack, soft-valve mitral stenosis. (a) Parasternal long axis view. (b) M-mode of mitral valve. (c) Correct assessment of the mitral surface area (MSA) using planimetry (1.54 cm²). (d) Incorrect assessment of the MSA using continuous Doppler (1.52 cm²). AO, aorta; LA, left atrium; LV, left ventricle; MO, mitral orifice; MS, mitral stenosis; RV, right ventricle.

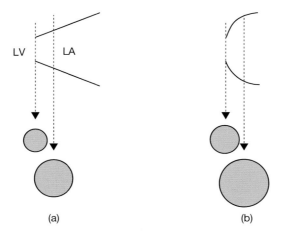

Figure 6.10   Morphological forms of the mitral stenosis: (a) funnel shape; (b) membrane shape. There is a risk of a clear overestimation of the mitral surface area using planimetry passing through the body of the mitral valve in the form of a membrane. LA, left atrium; LV, left ventricle.

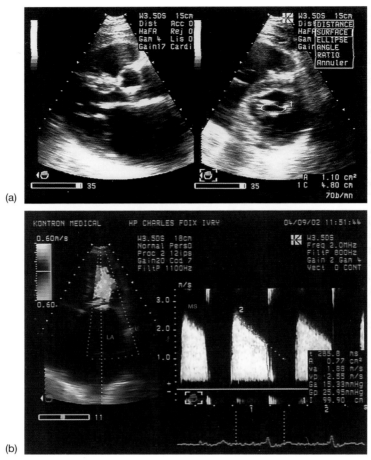

Figure 6.11   Tight mitral stenosis (MS) with clear remodelling of the subvalvular apparatus. The mitral surface area measured using planimetry (1.1 cm²) (a) is larger than that determined using continuous-wave Doppler (0.77 cm²) (b). LA, left atrium.

Non-linear decrease in velocity in mitral stenosis

This is a particular morphology of the Doppler curve: a biphasic slope with a steep, brief initial period, followed by a slower phase (Fig. 6.12). Given this ambiguity regarding which slope should be used, it is recommended that the PHT measurement is made using the second slope (Fig. 6.13). However, in the majority of patients, the deceleration slope is a straight line.

Flutters

Flutters may present pitfalls when using Hatle's method:

- Sinus tachycardia (> 100 beats/min) leads to an overestimation of the MSA by shortening the duration of the mitral E wave, and therefore the duration

---

Box 6.3   Pitfalls when using Hatle's method to measure the mitral surface area

- Imperfect definition of the spectral envelope
- Non-linear decrease in veocity in mitral stenosis
- Presence of flutters
- In associated haemodynamic conditions (aortic stenosis, aortic regurgitation, mitral regurgitation, filling problem, etc.)
- In older patients
- During physical exercise
- During mitral valvuloplasty as a result of the rapid increase in the end-diastolic pressure

---

of the PHT. The brevity of the descending slope of the E wave may make it difficult to measure the PHT. Likewise, a fusion of the E and A waves (telescoping) in less tight MS may impede measurement of the mitral slope.

- Atrial flutter can disrupt the deceleration slope of the mitral flow.
- Atrial fibrillation may be responsible for a variable PHT. In the case of short R–R intervals, the PHT is shortened. Averaging over 5 to 10 cardiac cycles is necessary in this situation.

Associated haemodynamic conditions

- AS, major AR and disorders of left ventricular compliance (cardiac regurgitation, restrictive cardiomyopathy, etc.). In these cases, shortening of the PHT is due to the more rapid fall of the transmitral gradient as a result of the elevation of the end-diastolic pressure of the LV. This leads to an overestimation of the actual MSA.

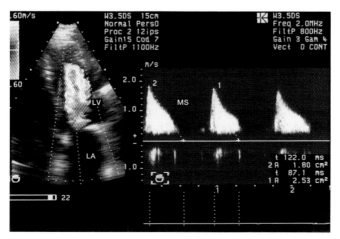

Figure 6.12   Mitral stenosis (MS) with a 'biphasic slope'. The mitral surface area measured using the initial slope (2.53 cm²) and the second slope (1.8 cm²) of the spectrum, recorded using continuous Doppler. LA, left atrium; LV, left ventricle.

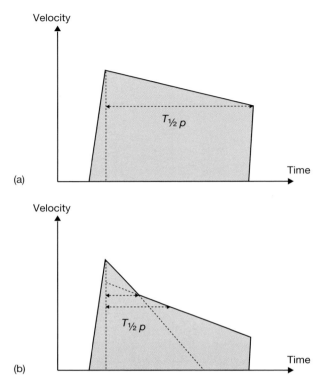

Figure 6.13   Measurement of the pressure half-time ($T_{1/2\,p}$) in cases of mitral stenosis (MS) with (a) linear and (b) non-linear deceleration slopes. There is a risk of overestimating MS when the measurement is made using the initial phase of the biphasic slope (b).

- Major mitral regurgitation and disorders of left ventricular relaxation (parietal hypertrophy, ischaemic cardiomyopathy, etc.). In these cases, a lengthening of the PHT increases the risk of underestimating the MSA.

Older patients
In certain older patients, Hatle's method leads to an overestimation of the MSA, which, apart from the above considerations, is due also to a reduction in left ventricular compliance.

Physical exercise
Physical exercise that modifies the pressure in the left atrium and the appearance of the mitral flow (shortened PHT) is also a possible pitfall of Hatle's method.

Following mitral valvuloplasty
Immediately after percutaneous mitral dilatation, the PHT values are responsible for an overestimation of the MSA. This phenomenon is linked to the sharp modifications in atrioventricular compliance postdilatation. Hatle's method must, therefore, not be used in the 48 hours following the dilatation procedure.

In practice
Planimetry is the preferred method in cases where there is satisfactory imaging, and Hatle's method is preferred in cases of a severely calcified mitral orifice, subvalvular stenosis or poor quality imaging. When there is a discrepancy between the results obtained using mitral planimetry and Hatle's method, it is necessary to resort to a third method (continuity equation). Finally, colour Doppler has a secondary role in assessing the tightness of the MS. It helps to position the Doppler beam in the central laminar part of the stenotic jet (the central core of the stenosis). Finally, Hatle's method is no longer considered valid for native mitral valves.

Pitfalls when using the continuity equation (Box 6.4)
The continuity equation uses the principle of conservation of mass, with the formula:

$$S_1 \times V_1 = S_2 \times V_2$$

where V_1 and V_2 are the subaortic and transvalvular stenotic velocities, and S_1 and S_2 are the aortic and subaortic (outflow) areas, respectively. The equation is based on the equality of the outputs:

- the aortic and mitral outputs in the case of MS
- the left ventricular outflow chamber output and the aortic orifice output in the case of AS.

Box 6.4   Pitfalls of the continuity equation when measuring the aortic surface area

Measurement of the subaortic diameter
- Inappropriate 2D cross-section
- Oblique angle of measurement
- Valvular or annular calcifications
- Subaortic septal rim
- Septal kinking

Measurement of the subaortic velocities
- Oblique apical 2D cross-section
- Incorrect positioning of the Doppler sample voume
- Inadequate quality of the spectrum
- Associated pathologies (aortic regurgitation, obstructive cardiomyopathy, atrial fibrillation)

Measurement of the stenotic velocities
- Poor alignment with the stenotic jet
- Inadequate quality of the spectrum
- Associated pathologies: obstructive cardiomyopathy, atrial fibrillation
- Confusion between the aortic stenosis flow and mitral regurgitation, tricuspid regurgitation or subaortic obstruction flows

Doppler TTE makes it possible to calculate the functional surface area of the stenotic orifice (mitral or aortic), which is equal to the output in the left ventricular outflow chamber divided by the velocity–time integral (VTI) of the trans-stenotic flow:

$$S_2 = \frac{S_1 \times V_1}{V_2}$$

This examination requires a high degree of technical rigour and precision of measurement in order to avoid the pitfalls of quantifying the valvular stenosis.

The following measurements are involved (Fig. 6.14):

- the subaortic diameter (D) making it possible to calculate the surface area of the left ventricular outflow chamber (S_1) by means of the formula:

$$S_1 = \pi \times D^2/4$$

- the subaortic velocities (V_1)
- the transvalvular stenotic velocities (V_2).

In practice, the maximum velocities and the VTI can be used interchangeably when calculating the aortic surface area.

Pitfalls when measuring the subaortic diameter

Incorrect use of the 2D apical cross-section centred on the aortic orifice
Imprecise measurement of the subaortic diameter using this approach is linked to the low lateral resolution of the ultrasonic waves in this view. The aortic orifice is approached in a tangential manner, and therefore there is a risk of underestimating the diameter of the left ventricular outflow chamber. For these reasons, the subaortic diameter should be measured in the longitudinal, parasternal cross-section, in systole, using the zoom and cine loop.

Poor visibility of the points of insertion of the aortic cusps
This problem is most often due either to insufficient patient echogenicity, or to valvular or annular calcifications masking the insertion of the semilunar cusps (Fig. 6.15).

Imprecise measurement of the subaortic diameter
Normally, this measurement should be carried out between the two points of insertion of the aortic cusps and in parallel with the plane of the valve. Care must be taken to measure the subaortic diameter with the greatest possible precision, since, if a mistake is made, the squaring of the diameter will modify the calculated valve surface area by the same amount. The following situations may be responsible for errors in measuring the subaortic diameter (Figs 6.16 and 6.17):

- the oblique view may falsely increase the value of the diameter
- the presence of a subaortic septal rim – the measurement should be taken downstream of the rim in order to avoid underestimating the diameter
- the existence of septal kinking – this abnormal kinking of the septum in relation to the aorta may disrupt the measurement of the subaortic diameter (risk of overestimation).

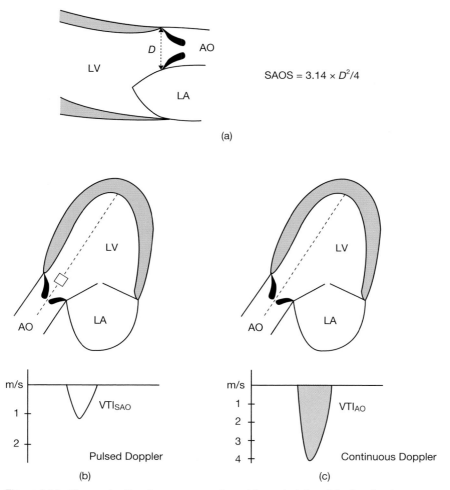

$$SAOS = 3.14 \times D^2/4$$

Figure 6.14   Three echo Doppler measurements enabling calculation of the functional surface area of the aortic orifice by means of the continuity equation. AO, aorta; D, diameter; LA, left atrium; LV, left ventricle; SAOS, subaortic surface; VTI_{AO}, aortic velocity–time integral; VTI_{SAO}, subaortic velocity–time integral.

In practice, the measurement of the left ventricular outflow chamber diameter should be repeated at least three times and the mean value calculated; any extreme, non-reproducible values should be eliminated.

The following formula offers an additional possibility for calculating the diameter of the subaortic diameter (D):

$$D = (0.01 \times \text{patient height in cm}) + 0.25$$

Values of D calculated using this formula are relatively reliable. However, use of the fixed value of 2 cm for the subaortic diameter should be avoided, as this is

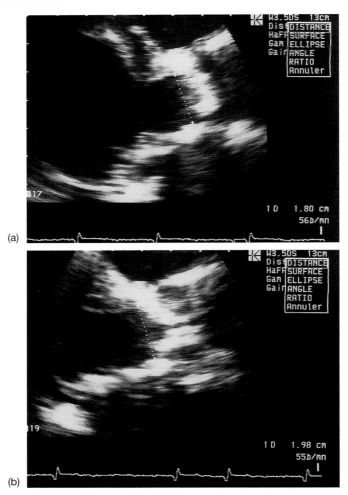

(a)

(b)

Figure 6.15 Aortic stenosis. Difficulty in precisely measuring the subaortic diameter when there is significant annular and valvular calcification. Values obtained from the same patient: (a) 1.8 cm and (b) 1.98 cm. Zoomed 2D images (longitudinal, parasternal cross-section).

a major source of errors. An incorrectly enlarged subaortic diameter will lead to an overestimation of the valve surface area (mitral or aortic) calculated using the continuity equation (Box 6.5). Conversely, a value for the subaortic diameter that is falsely too low will lead to an underestimation of the valve surface area.

Finally, in cases of AS where the measurement of the subaortic diameter is not possible via the transthoracic route, it is possible to quantify the stenosis using the permeability index. This may be done using the VTI ratio: subaortic VTI/transaortic VTI. This easily calculated parameter is independent of the cardiac output and its sensitivity is satisfactory, but its specificity remains poor.

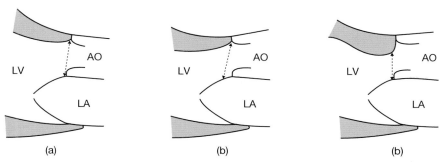

Figure 6.16 Measurements of the subaortic diameter when using 2D echocardiography and the longitudinal, parasternal cross-section. (a) Correct angle; (b) oblique angle overestimating the diameter; (c) angle underestimating the diameter in the case of a subaortic septal rim included in the measurement. AO, aorta; LA, left atrium; LV, left ventricle.

Box 6.5   Possible causes of overestimation of the aortic surface area calculated using the continuity equation

- Overestimation of the aortic diameter
- Overestimation of the subaortic velocity–time integral
- Underestimation of the transaortic velocity–time integral

In fact, a ratio of ≤ 0.25 identifies an aortic surface area of ≤ 0.75 cm² with a sensitivity of 92% and a specificity of 68%.

Finally, in an extreme diagnostic situation, the operator may resort to TEE to measure the subaortic diameter with greater precision.

Pitfalls when recording subaortic flows
Normally, these flows should be recorded using pulsed Doppler across the apical cross-section passing through the aortic root. It is important to be aware of the potential pitfalls of this technique (see Box 6.4).

Overly oblique view of the left ventricular outflow chamber
In order to minimize the angle between the Doppler beam and the subaortic flow, it is often necessary to move the echocardiographic probe towards the armpit of the patient being examined. This manipulation makes it possible to verticalize the outflow chamber and to obtain a better alignment of the Doppler beam with the aortic ejection flow.

Incorrect positioning of the Doppler sample volume in the left ventricular outflow chamber
In practice, the small Doppler sample volume (4–6 mm) should be positioned in the middle of the left ventricular outflow chamber, approximately 5 mm upstream of the aortic cusps, a position that corresponds fairly well with the level used for measuring the subaortic diameter in the parasternal view. Colour Doppler may

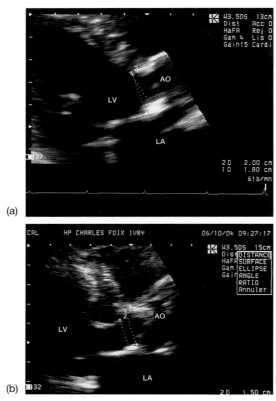

Figure 6.17 Aortic stenosis. Pitfalls in measuring the subaortic diameter using the longitudinal parasternal cross-section (zoomed images). (a) Oblique angle overestimating (2.0 cm) the actual diameter (1.8 cm). (b) Underestimation of the aortic diameter (1.5 cm) measured at the level of the subaortic septal rim. Correct value obtained downstream of the rim: 1.8 cm. AO, aorta; LA, left atrium; LV, left ventricle.

make it easier to locate the site of collection of the subaortic flow. This site usually corresponds to the small first aliasing zone (passage from blue to red) in the absence of low output. By modifying slightly the position of the Doppler sample volume in the outflow chamber, it is possible to optimize the collection of subaortic velocities. This process enables the operator to record subaortic flows integrally within the exclusively laminar zone, at the level of the vena contracta.

An underestimation of the subaortic velocities is due to the Doppler sample volume being too distant from the aortic valve. This leads to an underestimation of the valve surface area calculated using the continuity equation. Bringing the Doppler sample volume too close to the aortic orifice leads to a sharp enlargement of the spectrum linked to the entry into the acceleration zone of the ejection flow. This in turn leads to an overestimation of the subaortic velocities, and therefore to an erroneous increase in the valve surface area calculated using the continuity equation (Fig. 6.18).

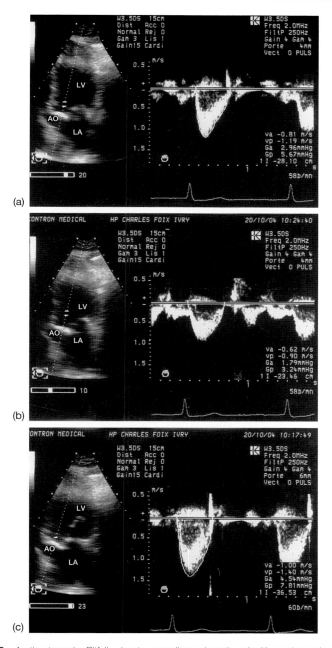

Figure 6.18   Aortic stenosis. Pitfalls due to recording subaortic velocities using pulsed Doppler; all views are in the same patient. (a) Correct recording site (velocity–time integral (VTI): 28 cm). (b) Incorrect site, too far from the aortic orifice (VTI underestimated: 23 cm). (c) Incorrect site, too close to the aortic orifice (VTI overestimated: 36 cm). AO, aorta; LA, left atrium; LV, left ventricle.

Poor quality of the subaortic spectrum recorded using pulsed Doppler
The poor quality of the subaortic spectrum recorded using pulsed Doppler renders the subaortic VTI measurement using planimetry imprecise. It is important to obtain a clear spectral envelope of the subaortic flows, with well-defined and homogenous contours, and without echoes within the spectrum. The presence of the aortic closing click is not a required condition for recording; this click is often muffled in the case of a tight AS. Finally, the measurement of the subaortic VTI should be done over at least three cycles and the mean value calculated.

Associated pathologies
Associated pathologies that render the recording of subaortic flows less reliable are:

- Major AR and obstructive cardiomyopathy, which increase the subaortic velocity. In effect, the continuity equation is not valid in the presence of a left intraventricular acceleration (above 1.5 m/s), as the subaortic velocity is no longer insignificant in this context. In this situation, the pulmonary output can be used to calculate the mitral valve surface area by means of the continuity equation.
- Atrial fibrillation, which leads to variable values of the subaortic VTI (Fig. 6.19). In this case planimetry should be used, taking the mean value of at least five consecutive cardiac cycles at relatively constant R–R intervals.

Finally, post-extrasystolic complexes should be avoided when measuring the subaortic VTI, as they lead to a post-extrasystolic increase in the subaortic flow.

Pitfalls when recording the stenotic flow
The transvalvular stenotic flow (mitral or aortic) is recorded using continuous Doppler. It is important to understand the pitfalls of this type of recording in order to avoid incorrect results (see Box 6.4).

Poor alignment of the Doppler beam with the stenotic flow
Poor alignment of the Doppler beam with the stenotic flow leads to an incomplete recording of the stenotic jet and a 'hoarse' and vibrant Doppler sound. It is therefore necessary to increase the number of echocardiographic views, especially when exploring AS. When done with care, it is possible to achieve correct alignment and to capture the maximum velocity of the stenosis. The pure and sharp acoustic signal indicates proper alignment. Prior localization of the stenotic flow using colour Doppler, wherein it is seen in the form of a mosaic, enables precise adjustment of the Doppler beam angle (Fig. 6.20).

Failure to use the 2 MHz, Pedoff-type, continuous, stand-alone Doppler probe (pen-shaped probe) without 2D imaging ('blind')
The great ease of manipulating of this probe allows for optimal alignment of the beam with the central jet of the stenosis. Poor alignment (above 20°) leads to a clear underestimation of the transvalvular VTI (Fig. 6.21), which leads to an overestimation of the valve surface area as calculated using the continuity equation (see Box 6.5).

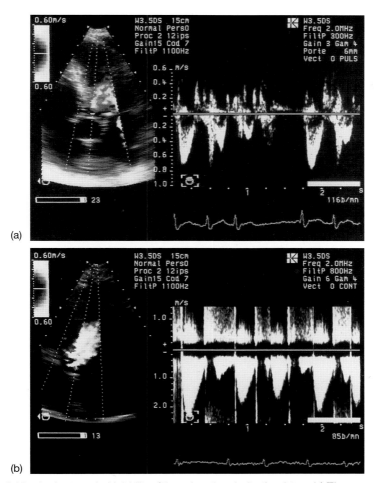

Figure 6.19   Aortic stenosis. Variability of the subaortic velocity–time integral (VTI) measured using pulsed Doppler (a) and of the transaortic VTI measured using continuous Doppler (b) in the case of continuous arrhythmia due to atrial fibrillation.

Failure to average the transvalvular velocity–time integral measurements
As with subaortic flows, it is recommended that at least three cardiac cycles in sinus rhythm are recorded, avoiding post-extrasystolic complexes, and the mean VTI value calculated. In the case of atrial fibrillation, VTI values from a minimum of five cycles should be averaged, due to the variability in the VTI of the stenotic flow during continuous arrhythmia (see Fig. 6.19).

Associated pathologies
Failure to use the continuity equation to calculate the MSA in the case of major AR (increase in the subaortic VTI) or MR (increase in the transmitral VTI) associated with MS.

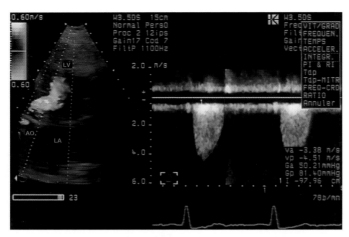

Figure 6.20 Aortic stenosis. Stenotic flow recorded using continuous Doppler coupled with 2D imaging. Perfect alignment of the Doppler beam over the stenotic flow is picked up in colour Doppler imaging. AO, aorta; LA, left atrium; LV, left ventricle.

Confusion between the flow in aortic stenosis and the flow in mitral regurgitation when using the Pedoff probe (Fig. 6.22)
Successive recording of one flow after another makes it possible to differentiate easily between the AS and MR flows. Other elements may help to identify the aortic ejection flow, which:

- begins after the QRS complex, observing the isovolumetric contraction time (the flow due to MR appears from the beginning of the isovolumic contraction phase, coinciding with the mitral closing click, and continues until the mitral opening click)
- is framed by the opening and closing clicks of the aortic valve
- is of shorter duration than MR
- is in continuity with a possible flow due to AR that has the characteristic appearance.

Confusion between the flow in aortic stenosis and the flow in tricuspid regurgitation when using the Pedoff probe (see Fig. 6.22)
The differentiation between these flows is much easier than that between the AS and MR flows. The maximum flow velocity in tricuspid regurgitation (TR) is generally lower than that in AS, except in cases of severe pulmonary hypertension, or in cases of non-tight AS. The flow time in TR is longer than that of the aortic flow.

Confusion between the flow in aortic stenosis and the flow in left ventricular dynamic obstruction
In order to differentiate between these flows, the operator must make use of echocardiographic imaging and continuous Doppler. The obstructive subaortic flow shows an acceleration crescendo during the systole, which has a character-

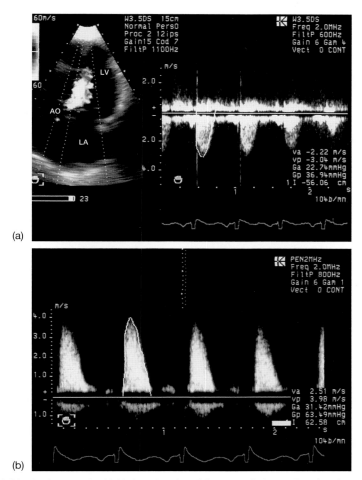

Figure 6.21 Aortic stenosis. (a) Underestimation of the transvalvular gradient (maximum gradient: 37 mmHg) calculated using the flow recorded with continuous Doppler coupled with 2D imaging (incorrect alignment). (b) Correct evaluation of the gradient (63 mmHg) obtained using the Pedoff probe, which enables good alignment with the stenotic jet (recorded in the same patient as in (a)). AO, aorta; LA, left atrium; LV, left ventricle.

istic sabre-shaped appearance (see Fig. 6.22). However, in cases of subvalvular obstruction associated with AS, the continuity equation is invalid, as the upstream velocity is no longer insignificant. The only usable method in this situation is planimetry of the aortic orifice.

Finally, in the presence of a subvalvular AS (e.g. in the membrane), the flow is difficult to differentiate from AS flow in continuous Doppler. In this case, pulsed or colour Doppler can be used to locate the site of the flow acceleration downstream of the aortic orifice.

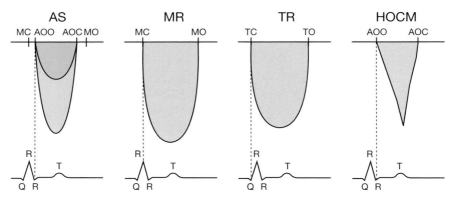

Figure 6.22 Differential diagnosis between aortic stenosis (AS) and mitral regurgitation (MR), and between tricuspid regurgitation (TR) and left intraventricular obstruction (hypertrophic obstructive cardiomyopathy (HOCM)), using flows recorded with continuous Doppler. Note the short ejection times (AS and HOCM) in relation to the length of MR or TR, and the isovolumetric contraction time (the period between the QRS wave and the start of the flow) in the case of AS or HOCM. AOC, aortic closing; AOO, aortic opening; MC, mitral closing; MO, mitral opening; TC, tricuspid closing; TO, tricuspid opening.

Pitfalls associated with aortic pseudostenosis

Aortic pseudostenosis is a tight AS (aortic surface area < 0.75 cm^2) with systolic dysfunction of the LV (ejection fraction $< 45\%$) and a low transvalvular gradient (average gradient < 30 mmHg). In this particular case, traditional echo Doppler does not allow differentiation between aortic pseudostenosis linked to left ventricular dysfunction with low output, and genuine tight AS with associated impaired ventricular function. Stress echocardiography under low doses of Dobutamine is very useful in this differential diagnosis. In fact, it makes it possible to identify the presence of a myocardial contractile reserve and to study the evolution of the gradients as well as the functional aortic surface area under stimulation. The presence of the contractile reserve is defined by an increase of 20% in the subaortic VTI or of 10% in the left ventricular ejection fraction.

The functional surface area increases by, on average, 0.1–0.3 cm^2 when the cardiac output is increased using Dobutamine, but the anatomical surface area

Table 6.2   The three types of haemodynamic response observed under Dobutamine in cases of low output AS

Response type	Output	Gradient	Surface area	Contractile reserve	Stenosis
I	↑	↑	Stable	Present	Tight
II	↑	Stable	↑	Present	Moderate
III	Stable	Stable	Stable	Absent	Undefined

↑, increased.

remains fixed. Three types of haemodynamic response are observed under Dobutamine, and these make it possible to define the therapeutic programme in the case of low-output AS (Table 6.2):

- Type I response, which reflects a genuinely tight AS with a contractile reserve that justifies surgical treatment of the stenosis.
- Type II response, which makes it possible to identify moderate AS (pseudo-tight in the basal state) associated with cardiomyopathy of other origin. It confirms the presence of an inotropic reserve. First-line medical treatment is necessary in this situation.
- Type III response, which makes it impossible to determine the tightness of the AS. This response shows the absence of a contractile reserve. In this case the therapeutic strategy is poorly defined, and should be discussed on a case-by-case basis.

Pitfalls associated with mitral stenosis when there is a discrepancy between clinical symptoms and echocardiographic data at rest

These are symptomatic patients with a mild MS, or asymptomatic patients with a tight stenosis. A discrepancy between symptoms and data justifies the use of exercise echocardiography to evaluate the functional significance of the MS. The evolution of the transmitral gradient and pulmonary pressures during exercise are analysed.

In exercise echocardiography, the criteria that indicate haemodynamic consequences of the MS are:

- an increase in the average gradient of > 15 mmHg at peak effort (or double the resting value)
- an increase in the systolic pulmonary arterial pressure of > 60 mmHg at peak stress.

The results of exercise echocardiography have considerable influence on the therapeutic treatment of these particular patients.

Pitfalls of the proximal isovelocity surface area (PISA) method

This method makes it possible to calculate the MSA on the basis of a convergence zone called the proximal isovelocity surface area (PISA) (Fig. 6.23). The convergence zone corresponds to an isovelocity zone of laminar flow, which converges towards the stenotic mitral orifice. This zone can be identified in the left atrium (LA) by using 2D colour Doppler (apical cross-section of the four chambers), by lowering the aliasing velocity (zero level of the velocity colour scale displaced upwards).

The MSA is calculated according to the formula:

$$MSA = \frac{2\pi r^2 V \times \alpha/180}{V_{max}}$$

where r is the radius of the convergence zone, V is the velocity of the convergence zone (aliasing velocity), $\alpha/180$ is the angle between the mitral valves and V_{max} is the maximum velocity of the transmitral flow.

The pitfalls of the PISA method when evauating the degree of MS are analogous to those encountered when evaluating MR using this method (see

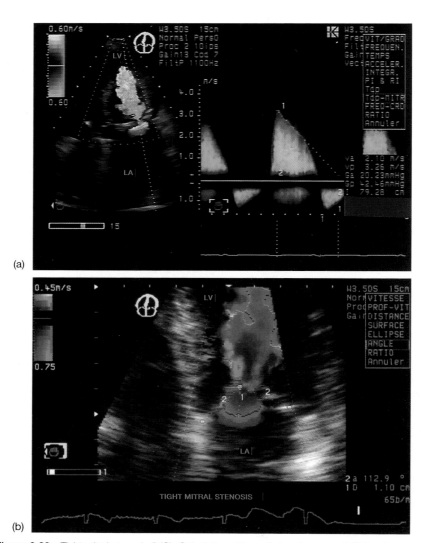

(a)

(b)

Figure 6.23 Tight mitral stenosis (MS). Calculation of the mitral surface area (MSA) using the PISA method (TTE). (a) Spectrum of the MS in continuous Doppler: maximum velocity (V_{max}) 326 cm/s. (b) Convergence zone in 2D colour Doppler: radius (r) 1.1 cm; aliasing velocity (V) 45 cm/s; angle $\alpha = 113°$.

$$MSA = \frac{2\pi r^2 V \times \alpha/180}{V_{max}} = \frac{(2 \times 3.14) \times 1.1^2 \times 45 \times 113/180}{326} = 0.66 \text{ cm}^2$$

LA, left atrium; LV, left ventricle.

page 86). As far as MS is concerned, neglect of the correction factor ($\alpha/180$), which takes into account the angle of the funnel formed by the mitral valves, leads to overestimation of the MS.

PITFALLS DUE TO THE CHOICE OF THRESHOLD VALUES FOR VALVULAR STENOSIS

The exact values that make it possible to identify a tight valvular stenosis (MS or AS) from echo Doppler measurements (average gradient, valve surface area) are, in the author's experience, relatively variable. In practice, the threshold values summarized in Table 6.3 are generally used. Of course, the severity criteria based on the measurement of the transvalvular gradient are valid in the case of normal left ventricular systolic function.

It is desirable to relate the valve surface area calculated using echo Doppler (cm^2) to the body surface area of the subject examined (m^2). This indexing of the stenotic surface area enables the calculation to be refined and the results to be interpreted at the level of the individual. Monitoring of the valvular stenosis by means of repeated examinations is also improved.

Finally, a permeability index below 0.25 is suggestive of a tight AS. Nevertheless, this value is less reliable than the measure of aortic surface area in judging the severity of a stenosis.

PITFALLS DUE TO THE HAEMODYNAMIC CONSEQUENCES OF VALVULAR STENOSIS

The pitfalls due to the haemodynamic consequences associated with MS (dilatation of the left atrium, interatrial thrombus, pulmonary hypertension) or AS (parietal hypertrophy, left ventricular dysfunction) are discussed on page 25.

VALVULAR LEAKS

The pitfalls encountered in the diagnosis of MR or AR are associated with:

- confusion between ultrasound artefacts and small valvular leaks
- difficulty in distinguishing between physiological and pathological leaks
- determining the aetiology of the leaks

Table 6.3   Echo Doppler severity criteria for mitral stenosis and aortic stenosis

Stenosis type	Average gradient	Valve surface area
Tight mitral stenosis	> 10 mmHg	< 1.5 cm² (< 1.0 cm²/m²)
Tight aortic stenosis	> 50 mmHg	< 0.7 cm² (< 0.45 cm²/m²)

- quantifying the degree of valvular regurgitation
- evaluating the haemodynamic consequences of leaks.

CONFUSION BETWEEN ULTRASOUND ARTEFACTS AND SMALL VALVULAR LEAKS

Ultrasound artefacts that simulate a small valvular leak, particularly of the mitral valve, are caused by the valve closing and suddenly stopping the flow upstream of the orifice. This stoppage gives rise to a discrete decrease in blood flow, which is manifested in colour Doppler as a central subvalvular microzone of the opposite colour to that of the valvular flow, without aliasing and without turbulence (false retrograde flow). In pulsed Doppler this phenomenon is manifested as an increase in noise associated with the valve closing (dense, enlarged line) (Fig. 6.24).

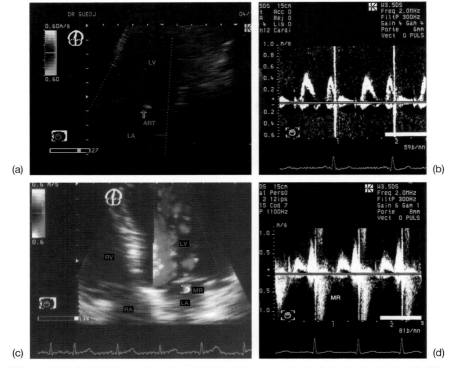

(a)   (b)

(c)   (d)

Figure 6.24   (a, b) Ultrasound artefact (ART) simulating a small mitral valve leak, obtained in 2D colour Doppler (blue microspot) and in pulsed Doppler (strengthening of the mitral closing click). (c, d) Tiny mitra regurgitation (MR) visualized in 2D colour Doppler (aliased turbulent jet) and in pulsed Doppler (early systolic regurgitation). LA, left atrium; LV, left ventricle; RA, right atrium; RV, right ventricle.

A genuine valvular leak is due to the absence of watertightness of the valve. A small leak corresponds to a low volume of regurgitant blood through the orifice, which is expressed in colour Doppler as a small, central or eccentric, aliased and turbulent subvalvular zone. The small convergence zone (zone of laminar flow, which converges at the leaking orifice) may also be identified (Fig. 6.25). Pulsed Doppler records the larger or smaller regurgitant flow that appears either side of the zero line (aliasing phenomenon). Continuous Doppler makes it possible to record the regurgitant flows, which are usually of low velocity, in a more or less integral fashion.

The elements of the echo Doppler image that make it possible to distinguish ultrasound artefacts from genuine small valvular leaks are summarized in Table 6.4.

DISTINGUISHING BETWEEN PHYSIOLOGICAL AND PATHOLOGICAL LEAKS

The diagnosis of a valvular leak is carried out clinically by means of auscultation, but in cases where the murmur is very weak or inaudible, Doppler echocardiography can be used to confirm the existence of a tiny valvular leak. In fact, minuscule valvular leaks are common in normal subjects (Fig. 6.26), and are considered to be physiological and commonplace. Colour Doppler has made it possible to recognize the high frequency of these leaks at the level of the right heart in a healthy heart (Table 6.5). Technical progress in colour Doppler has also made it possible to trace physiological leaks in the left heart in healthy subjects under 50 years old. These leaks usually occur at the level of the mitral valve. What is known as physiological MR is observed in more than one in two cases in young, healthy volunteers. In contrast, the presence of a physiological aortic leak is exceptional. Valvular leaks in the left heart increase in frequency

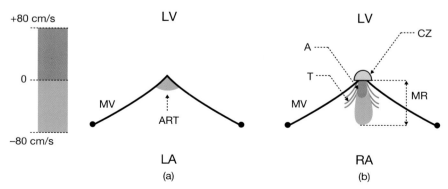

Figure 6.25   Differential diagnosis. (a) Ultrasound artefact (ART) simulating mitral regurgitation: the mitral valve (MV) is watertight, and the artefact is situated just below the valvular coaptation (blue area); the blood flow is non-aliased and non-turbulent. (b) True MR: there is incomplete closure of the mitral valve; the MR jet (blue area) is aliased (A, red area) and turbulent (T, green lines), and there is a convergence zone (CZ, yellow area). LA, left atrium; LV, left ventricle.

Table 6.4   Elements of echo Doppler images that make it possible to distinguish between ultrasound artefacts and actual small valvular leaks

Element	False leak	Actual leak
Source	Ultrasound artefact	Non-watertight valve
Mechanism	Blood flow stoppage	Blood regurgitation
Colour Doppler	*Subvalvular microzone*	
	Central	Central or eccentric
	Non-aliased	Aliased
	Non-turbulent	Turbulent
	Convergence zone	
	Absent	Present
Pulsed Doppler	Strengthened valve closing click	Bidirectional spectrum of regurgitant flow
Continuous Doppler	No useful signal	Monodirectional spectrum of regurgitant flow

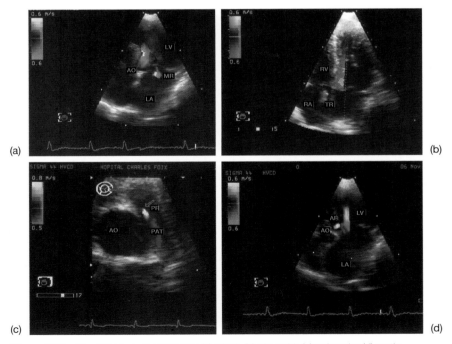

Figure 6.26   Physiological valvular leaks: (a) mitral; (b) tricuspid; (c) pulmonic; (d) aortic. AO, aorta; AR, aortic regurgitation; LA, left atrium; LV, left ventricle; MR, mitral regurgitation; PAT, pulmonary arterial trunk; PR, pulmonic regurgitation; RA, right atrium; RV, right ventricle; TR, tricuspid regurgitation.

Table 6.5 Frequency of physiological regurgitation

Site of regurgitation	Frequency (%)
Tricuspid	52–100
Pulmonic	22–100
Mitral	22–61
Aortic	0–6

with age due to cardiac ageing. They are also more common in athletes as a result of the modification of the heart geometry. In general, physiological leaks are small (< 1 cm²) and show little aliasing in colour Doppler. They are characterized by the absence of anomalies in the valve texture.

In practice, imaging a physiological TR or pulmonic regurgitation (PR) using continuous Doppler is useful for calculating the pulmonary arterial pressures. The progression over time of physiological leaks is little understood. Finally, the risk of endocarditis complicating these physiological leaks seems to be very low.

PITFALLS WHEN DIAGNOSING THE AETIOLOGY OF VALVULAR LEAKS

These pitfalls most often concern the diagnosis of three pathologies that may be responsible for a valvular regurgitation:

- mitral valve prolapse (MVP)
- infective endocarditis
- aortic dissection (see page 207).

Pitfalls when diagnosing mitral valve prolapse
TTE is a determining examination in the diagnosis of MVP, the most common valvulopathy in the population.

Pitfalls of M-mode echocardiography
Monodimensional M-mode echocardiography provides the classical and historical criteria for MVP, which are (Figs 6.27 and 6.28):

- a cup-shaped, end-systolic posterior displacement (> 2 mm) of the mitral echo
- a hammock-shaped holosystolic posterior displacement (> 3 mm) of the mitral echo.

The most specific picture of a prolapse is the end-systolic cup shape. The hammock-shaped picture of a prolapse is more common (60% of cases), but its specificity is markedly lower. M-mode echocardiography is unreliable in diagnosing MVP as it describes mitral movements in relation to a fixed point (the thoracic wall). A false appearance of a prolapse may thus arise when the whole of the mitral apparatus moves away from the probe without any genuine move-

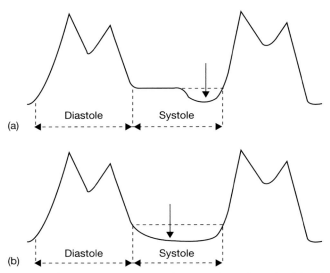

Figure 6.27   Images of mitral valve prolapse in M-mode echocardiography: (a) end-systolic cup shape; (b) holosystolic hammock shape.

ment of the valves in relation to the mitral annulus. In reality, M-mode echocardiography gives rise to numerous false-negative and false-positive diagnoses of MVP. Moreover, it does not allow exact identification of the prolapsed valve or assessment of the degree of systolic recoil in the LA.

Errors in diagnosing MVP when using M-mode echocardiography are:

- Technical problems:
  - a tangential M-mode view will underestimate the systolic recoil of the small mitral valve in particular
  - an ultrasound probe positioned too high over the thorax may give rise to an erroneously hammock-shaped image in a normal subject
  - poor lateral resolution of the ultrasound beam, reflecting off a particularly reflective surface area of the prolapsed valve, will give rise to an M-mode image that is limited to the multiple mitral echoes and echoes superimposed during systole, which do not contribute to the diagnosis of prolapse.
- Failure to recognize the prolapse of the lateral scallops of the small mitral valve. In fact, only the median scallop of the small valve is identifiable in M-mode echocardiography when using the traditional projection.
- Poor image specificity of the hammock-shaped prolapse. A falsely hammock-shaped MVP can be observed in a number of situations (Box 6.6).

Pitfalls of two-dimensional echocardiography
Two-dimensional echocardiography occupies a primary position in the diagnosis of MVP. It allows the diagnosis of a prolapse to be confirmed when M-mode

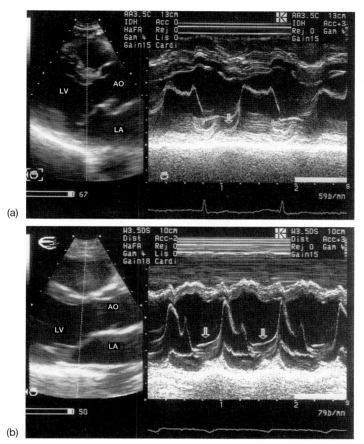

Figure 6.28   Images of mitral valve prolapse in M-mode echocardiography: (a) end-systolic cup shape; (b) holosystolic hammock shape. AO, aorta; LA, left atrium; LV, left ventricle.

Box 6.6   Causes of a falsely hammock-shaped mitral vave prolapse in M-mode echocardiography

- Hyperkinetic syndromes (fever, haemodialysis, etc.)
- Abundant pericardial effusion
- During ventricular extrasystoles
- Under administration of pharmacodynamic agents (glyceryl trinitrate, amyl nitrate, etc.)
- During a Valsalva manoeuvre

---

echocardiography cannot do so. Nonetheless, this technology can be responsible for false diagnoses of prolapse as a result of the following pitfalls (Box 6.7).

Box 6.7   Causes of false diagnosis of prolapse with 2D echocardiography

- Inappropriate choice of the 2D projection
- Atrioventricular plane created in the apical cross-section
- Defined saddle shape of the mitral annulus
- Poor definition of the plane of the mitral annulus
- Imprecise visualization of the valve coaptation
- Failure to respect the quantitative diagnostic criteria (see Table 6.6)

Inappropriate choice of the 2D projection

Two 2D views that allow echocardiographic diagnosis of MVP are commonly used: the parasternal, longitudinal cross-section of the heart and the apical cross-section of the four cardiac chambers.

Looking for a prolapse in an apical cross-section is responsible for a large number of false-positive diagnoses, and this has led to an overestimation of the frequency of the condition. In fact, an image of an MVP can be artificially induced in this view by using an excessively large angle between the ultrasound beam and the atrioventricular plane (Fig. 6.29).

Moreover, the defined saddle shape of the mitral annulus (parabolic hyperbole) can be responsible for a false appearance of a prolapse in the apical view in a normal subject. For these reasons, the echocardiographic diagnosis of MVP should be carried out using the longitudinal parasternal cross-section, which is considered to be the most reliable reference view (Fig. 6.30).

Failure to observe the rules for imaging a prolapse in the 2D mode

When studying a prolapse using 2D echocardiography in real time, it is necessary to beware of the misleading appearance of the image in movement. The diagnosis of MVP should be made using a frozen image, and preferably using the zoom and cine mode. Next, a virtual line is traced at the level of the mitral annulus (the reference point for the prolapse). This technique rests on an implicit hypothesis: i.e. that the mitral annulus is flat. However, it is possible to create an appearance of a prolapse in the apical cross-section without seeing the prolapse in the longitudinal cross-section perpendicular to it. This discrepancy occurs when the mitral annulus is saddle shaped, i.e. when its highest points are located anteriorly (subaortic) and posteriorly (Fig. 6.31). These are the points visualized in the longitudinal, parasternal cross-section. A systolic valvular movement visualized only in the apical cross-section is, therefore, the consequence of a normal valve geometry, without actual displacement of the mitral valves above the structure of the mitral annulus. The three-dimensional reconstruction of the mitral valve validates this geometric hypothesis (Fig. 6.32).

However, the correct definition of the plane of the mitral annulus may be difficult in the long axis, parasternal projection, as the mitral annulus, which is particularly hyperkinetic, may move during systole towards the LV. Finally, the diagnosis of an MVP using 2D echocardiography requires perfect definition of

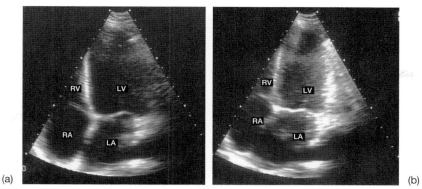

Figure 6.29   Normal subject: (a) apical cross-section of the four chambers correctly recorded (no mitral valve prolapse); (b) false appearance of an MVP artificially obtained due to atrioventricular plane. LA, left atrium; LV, left ventricle; RA, right atrium; RV, right ventricle.

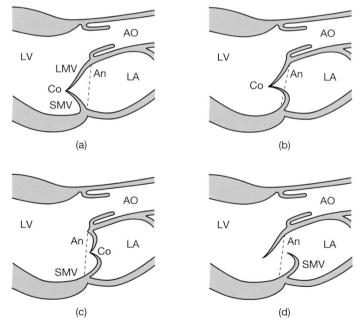

Figure 6.30   Appearance of the mitral valve in longitudinal, parasternal cross-section, during systole. (a) Normal image with the valvular coaptation (Co) situated in the foreground of the plane of the mitral annulus (An). (b) Ballooning of the small mitral valve (SMV). (c) Prolapse of both mitral valves. (d) Ruptured chordae with eversion of the SMV in the left atrium (LA). AO, aorta; LMV, large mitral valve; LV, left ventricle.

the point of systolic coaptation of the mitral valves, another reference point for the prolapse.

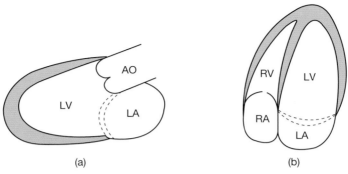

Figure 6.31 Morphological appearance of a saddle-shaped mitral annulus as imaged in: (a) the longitudinal, parasternal cross-section; (b) the apical cross-section of the four chambers. AO, aorta; LA, left atrium; LV, left ventricle; RA, right atrium; RV, right ventricle.

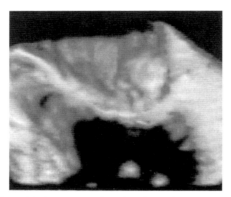

Figure 6.32 Three-dimensional reconstruction of a mitral valve proplapse in the atrial view.

Failure to observe the echocardiographic criteria for diagnosing a mitral valve prolapse

The term 'mitral valve prolapse' infers the existence of an abnormal movement of the mitral valve during systole in relation to a reference structure – the mitral annulus (see Fig. 6.30).

In order to confirm the pathological nature of an MVP using echocardiography, three elements must be taken into account:

- the degree of systolic movement of the mitral valve in the left atrium
- the degree of valvular dystrophy
- the existence and severity of the mitral leak.

The degree of valvular movement is assessed by the recoil of the systolic coaptation point of the mitral valves in relation to the plane of the mitral annulus.

The echocardiographic criteria currently proposed for securing the diagnosis of what is known as 'classic MVP' (Barlow's disease) are:

- the systolic protrusion of one or both mitral valves into the left atrium behind the plane of the mitral valve
- a systolic recoil of the coaptation point of the mitral valves by > 2 mm below the plane of the mitral annulus, with the valvular coaptation maintained
- an abnormal thickening of the mitral valve (maximum valve thickness of at least 5 mm).

'Non-classic valve prolapse' is the term used when there is a valve movement of > 2 mm during systole, with a maximum valve thickness of < 5 mm (Table 6.6). The term 'mitral ballooning' (a smaller echocardiographic shape than for prolapse) is reserved for shapes where the valvular recoil is < 2 mm or the valvular coaptation remains higher than the plane of the mitral annulus (see Figs 6.30 and 6.33). In this case there is neither abnormal valve thickening nor significant MR. Such an appearance should be considered a morphological variant of the normal mitral valve:

- in young normal subjects up to the age of 18 years (ballooning is noted in approximately 25% of cases)
- in normal subjects under certain haemodynamic conditions (hypovolaemia, hyperadrenergy).

Failure to observe the echocardiographic criteria for a diagnosis of prolapse, which have been recently redefined, may lead to an incorrect or mistaken diagnosis of an MVP.

Imprecision in locating a mitral valve prolapse

Two-dimensional echocardiography makes it possible directly to identify the prolapsed valve, and to specify the location and extent of the prolapse. This information is particularly useful in assessing the patient for potential conservative surgery.

However, there are certain pitfalls in determining the location of the prolapse, relating to:

- the mono- or bivalvular nature of the prolapse
- partial prolapse of the mitral valve involving an isolated valve segment
- commissural prolapse.

In order to avoid these pitfalls, a complete anatomical and functional analysis of the whole of the mitral apparatus is necessary. This should be carried out systematically transthoracically, with the transoesophageal route recommended

Table 6.6 Echocardiographic criteria for the diagnosis of classical and non-classical mitral valve prolapse and mitral ballooning

Criterion	Prolapse		Ballooning
	Classical	Non-classical	
Systolic recoil	> 2 mm	> 2 mm	< 2 mm
Valve thickness	> 5 mm	< 5 mm	Normal

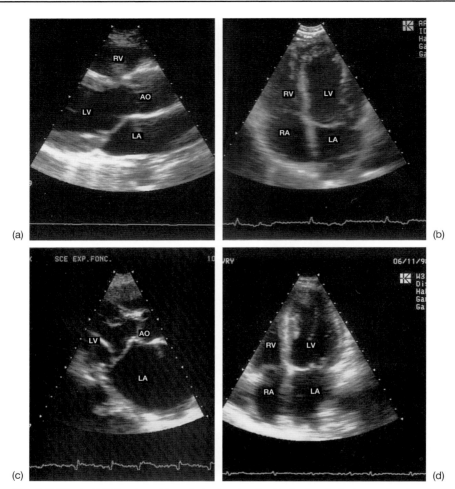

Figure 6.33   (a, b) Ballooning of the mitral valve visualized in the longitudinal, parasternal and apical cross-sections of the four chambers. (c, d) Prolapse of both mitral valves seen in the same cross-sections as (a, b). AO, aorta; LA, left atrium; LV, left ventricle; RA, right atrium; RV, right ventricle.

only in cases of complicated shapes or in the context of a preoperative check-up (Fig. 6.34). A standardized segmentation of the mitral valve facilitates a precise description of the valvular lesions. Use of multiple echocardiographic projections allows for an exploration of all the mitral segments and the commissures (see Fig. 6.2).

However, comparison of the echocardiographic images with anatomical data reveals certain differences regarding the location of the prolapse. In fact, 2D echocardiography may show a prolapse of both mitral valves, despite degenerative anatomical lesions affecting only one valve. This phenomenon can be

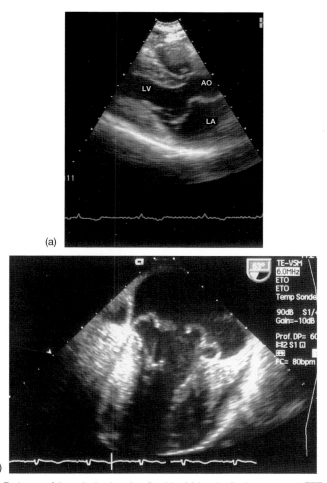

Figure 6.34   Prolapse of the mitral valve visualized in: (a) longitudinal, parasternal TTE cross-section; (b) multiplanar TEE cross-section. AO, aorta; LA, left atrium; LV, left ventricle.

explained by the physiological mechanism of the closure of the mitral valves. The mitral leaflets come together during ventricular systole, and therefore the prolapse of one valve encourages the recoil of the other. It seems that a 'functional' recoil, of variable size, of the opposing valve often accompanies the prolapse of the valve altered by degeneration.

Incomplete appreciation of mitral valve thickening

Abnormal mitral valve thickening is a reflection of the myxomatous infiltration of the spongy layer of the mitral valve. This myxomatous degeneration of the valve tissue is confirmed in echocardiography by the existence of the following elements:

- a maximum valve thickness ≥ 5 mm, as measured using M-mode imaging midsystole, in the longitudinal, parasternal cross-section
- clubbing (golf-club shape) of the end of the myxomatous valve
- increased motion of the valve affected by degeneration.

A thorough study of the whole of the mitral valve apparatus from various views is necessary in order to confirm the dystrophic injury.

On M-mode images myxomatous degeneration appears as thickened mitral echoes, called 'redundant', sometimes fluttering. In 2D echocardiography, 'myxomatous swellings' appended to the valve are clearly visible in the transverse, parasternal cross-section (Fig. 6.35). During diastole, the large mitral valve, which is flaccid and distended as a result of the dystrophy, undergoes a characteristic deformation into the shape of a helmet. Sometimes, the myxomatous thickening of the mitral valve is such that they appear on the image to be vegetations or even a myxoma. The chordae can be lengthened and thinned or, more often, thickened. A rupture of the chordae is also possible. The mitral annulus is more or less dilated.

Echocardiographic detection of myxomatous degeneration of the mitral valve makes it possible to confirm Barlow's disease and to identify patients with a high risk of complications.

Finally, in older patients, Barlow's disease must be distinguished from fibroelastic degeneration, which is often complicated by a mitral valve eversion through rupture of the chordae. However, in these particular dystrophic forms, there is no abnormal valve thickening; rather, the mitral valves are fine and transparent (Box 6.8).

Failure to identify ruptured chordae

The echocardiographic identification of ruptured chordae associated with MVP is a function of the number and the location on the valves of the ruptures. The rupture generally involves the chordae of the small mitral valve.

A positive diagnosis of ruptured chordae rests on examination using 2D echocardiography. It requires the association of two criteria:

- the absence of coaptation of the mitral valves during systole
- systolic eversion in the left atrium of the free end of the valve with the ruptured chordae (see Figs 6.30 and 6.36).

The term 'flail' corresponds to the most serious and diffuse form of prolapse, which is often complicated by ruptured chordae.

Box 6.8 Causes of abnormal thickening of the mitral valve	
• Myxomatous degeneration	• Valvular calcification
• Fibroelastic degeneration	• Vegetations adhering to the valve
• Post-rheumatic thickening	• Myxoma or other valvular tumour

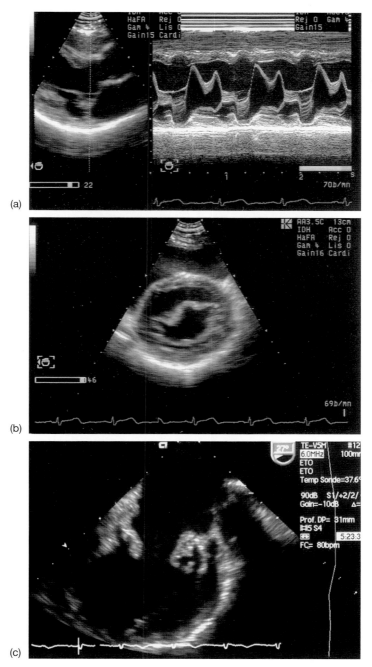

Figure 6.35 Barlow's disease. Thick, myxomatous appearance of a prolapsed mitral valve: (a) M-mode TTE projection; (b) TTE 2D transverse, parasternal projection; (c) multiplanar TEE.

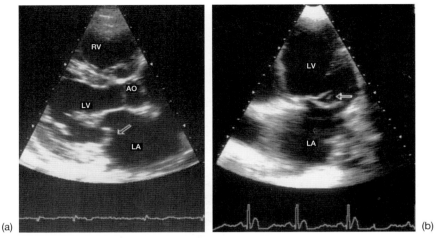

Figure 6.36 Chordal rupture of the small mitral valve as identified in the longitudinal, parasternal cross-section (a) and the apical cross-section of the four chambers (b). AO, aorta; LA, left atrium; LV, left ventricle; RV, right ventricle.

The echocardiographic pitfalls that may be encountered in diagnosing ruptured chordae are:

- Distinguishing between an extreme elongation of the chordae and ruptured chordae (which give similar echocardiographic images) is practically impossible. Moreover, elongations and ruptures of the chordae can coexist in the same patient. The direct visualization of a piece of ruptured chorda attached to the valve and flail in the ventricular chamber is rare but possible, particularly in TEE. This image should not be confused with a valvular vegetation.
- It is difficult to detect ruptures to the principal basal and paracommissural chordae when using TTE. However, such ruptures can be detected markedly better using multiplanar TEE.

Finally, it is necessary to distinguish between genuine degenerative MVP (Barlow's disease) and MVP 'secondary' to various cardiac pathologies (chronic rheumatic endocarditis, ischaemic cardiopathy, asymmetric septal hypertrophy, dilated cardiomyopathy, interatrial communication, cardiac trauma). This type of MVP is a semiological epiphenomenon in the evolution of these conditions.

Pitfalls when diagnosing infective endocarditis

Echocardiography plays a fundamental role in diagnosing infective endocarditis, as it provides major diagnostic elements. The pitfalls associated with the echocardiographic imaging of endocarditis principally concern the visualization of valvular vegetations and the detection of destructive lesions. In all cases the interpretation of the echocardiographic images must take into account the clinical context.

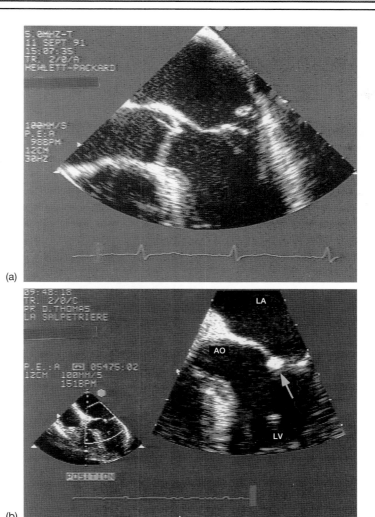

Figure 6.37   Mitral endocarditis explored in TEE. (a) A pedunculated mobile vegetation attached to the small mitral valve. (b) 'Organized', longstanding mitral vegetation. AO, aorta; LA, left atrium; LV, left ventricle.

Diagnostic pitfalls due to endocardial vegetations

Classically, the diagnosis of vegetations rests on the detection with 2D echo-cardiography of a mass of abnormal echoes appended to the valve or to an endocardial structure that is round or oblong, more or less mobile or even pedunculated, and brighter than the adjacent tissue (Figs 6.37 and 6.38).

The sensitivity of TTE in the detection of vegetations is of the order of 70%, as opposed to > 90% for TEE; both techniques have similarly high specificities.

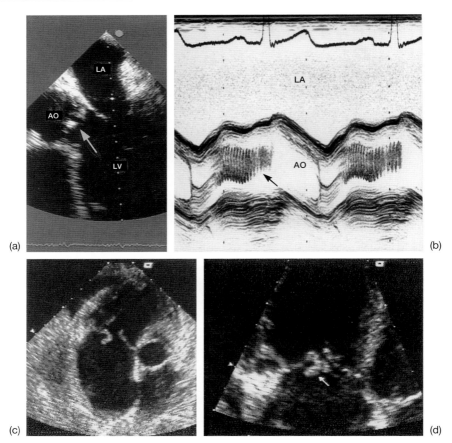

Figure 6.38   (a, b) A small aortic vegetation viewed in TEE (2D and M-mode); there is a 'hairy' appearance during diastole. (c, d) A large pedunculated tricuspid vegetation, viewed in TTE. AO, aorta; LA, left atrium; LV, left ventricle.

The pitfalls of echocardiographic imaging, particularly in the transthoracic projection, in making a positive diagnosis of vegetations are as follows.

Valvular vegetations with a thickness < 3 mm
Vegetations of this size often go unnoticed in echocardiography, as the echocardiographic resolution is not sufficient to detect their presence. Moreover, the adjustment of the gain should be correct, as too low a gain may cause a poorly echoic vegetation to disappear from the image.

Absence of vegetations during examination
The absence of vegetative lesions on echocardiographic examination does not indicate the absence of an endocarditis. In fact, the echocardiographic appearance of vegetations may be delayed in the evolution of the endocarditis in

relation to the clinical presentation. This is a frequent cause of false-negative results (Box 6.9). Therefore, when there is a strong diagnostic reason to suspect endocarditis, it is necessary to repeat the examination if the echocardiographic result is negative.

Distinction between a vegetation and other valvular lesions

The echocardiographic distinction between a vegetation and other valvular lesions is sometimes difficult, or even impossible. Questionable echocardiographic images, suggesting a vegetation, may be observed in a patient with suspected endocarditis. The most common causes of orientation errors (false-positive results) are summarized in Box 6.10. They arise in particular when, due to underlying cardiac pathology, the valves are thickened, fibrosed, calcified or myxomatous.

The difficulty in achieving a diagnosis of endocarditis arises, in particular, in patients presenting with a dystrophic condition of the mitral valve when there is also an associated rupture of the chordae.

In all these pathological situations, the differential diagnosis is made by referring to the clinical context. However, if there is the slightest doubt, there should be no hesitation in repeating the echocardiographic examination, and all the more so if the clinical profile is highly suggestive of endocarditis. TEE can make a useful contribution in these cases.

Distinction between an active vegetation and a sterile or treated vegetation

Distinguishing echocardiographically between a bacteriologically active vegetation and a sterile or treated vegetation is impossible. Likewise, no correlation has been found between the echocardiographic appearance of vegetations and

---

Box 6.9   Causes of false-negative results in the echocardiographic diagnosis of vegetations

Technical failures
- Observation conditions
- Quality of the equipment
- Technique used (transthoracic or transoesophageal, etc.)

Vegetations
- < 3 mm in size
- Absent in the initial clinical phase of the endocarditis
- Invisible due to their atypical location
- Masked by a mechanical valve prosthesis, particularly aortic
- Occurring on the cavitary thrombus
- Impossible to find due to embolic migration
- Multivalvular, proliferated or in multiple locations (orifices and walls)

the nature of the infecting organism, apart from yeasts, which give rise to large, highly echoic vegetations.

Non-inflammatory aetiology of vegetations
Generally, vegetations are of bacterial origin and are due to inflammation of the endocardium. The presence of non-infective vegetations has been noted in Libman–Sack endocarditis or marastic endocarditis. This type of vegetation can also cause false-positive echocardiographic results.

Atypical location of vegetations
Typically, the vegetations are initially valvular, and are most often located on the ventricular surface of the aortic valve and the auricular surface of the mitral valve. Other, atypical, locations (e.g. mural) are much less common (Box 6.11).

Vegetations on healthy valves
The presence of vegetations on healthy valves is exceptional. This diagnostic element should be borne in mind when interpreting questionable echocardiographic images. In general, vegetations almost always attach themselves to a valve that is already pathological. Very often, the valve is the site of a leak.

Paucity of clinical indications of endocarditis
The paucity of clinical cardiac indications of endocarditis should reinforce the echocardiographic search for vegetations. In this context, echocardiography becomes extremely important in the diagnosis. A thorough examination of the vegetations is therefore crucial. Recourse to TEE is still often essential.

Identification of vegetations on mechanical prostheses
The echocardiographic identification of vegetations on mechanical prostheses can be difficult. In fact, a strong reflection from the prosthetic material can mask the vegetating lesion. Likewise, it is almost impossible to distinguish between a vegetation and an infected thrombus attached to the valve prosthesis, all the more so because these two complications may be associated.

Persistence of vegetations
The persistence of vegetations long after clinical healing of the endocarditis is frequently noted. In fact, vegetations may remain similar to their initial form. These residual vegetations often pose a problem of differential diagnosis in the case of relapsing endocarditis or a recurrence of high temperature over the course of an endocarditis.

Finally, vegetations may organize in the long term by becoming fibrosed or even calcified (see Fig. 6.37). This situation may also make it difficult to diagnose a relapse.

Sudden disappearance of a vegetating lesion
The sudden disappearance of a vegetating lesion during the evolution of the endocarditis may be observed using echocardiography. This situation occurs when there is embolic migration of the vegetation, and is due to the friability

---

Box 6.10   Causes of false-positive results in the echocardiographic diagnosis of vegetations

- Valvular thickening as a secondary consequence of the inflammatory process (post-rheumatic nodules)
- 'Nodular', localized, valvular calcifications
- Myxomatous degeneration of the valve at the prolapse
- Partial rupture of the mitral chordae
- Valvular laceration
- Certain valvular or juxtavalvular masses, such as myxomas, papillary pseudo-tumours of the valves, pedunculated thrombi, Lambl excrescences (valvular flaps)
- Marastic vegetations (non-bacterial thrombotic endocarditis) or verrucous Libman–Sachs vegetations
- Degeneration of a bioprostheses
- Certain thrombi on valvular prostheses
- Fibrous deposits, fibrin strands

Box 6.11   Atypical locations of vegetations

- The septal interventricular endocardium (obstructive hypertrophic cardiomyopathy, interventricular communication)
- The mitral chordae
- A calcified mitral annulus
- The sinus of Valsalva
- The right heart (pacing wire, venous catheter, drug abuse, etc.)
- A myocardial abscess, particularly septal
- An intracardiac or intra-aortic prosthesis
- A complex congenital cardiac pathology (Fallot's tetralogy, arterial canal, aortic coarctation)
- A cardiac graft

---

of the vegetating mass, particularly if it is recent. The risk of embolism increases according with the size (diameter > 10 mm) and/or mobility of the vegetation, and whether it is increasing in volume. Fungal endocarditis is characterized by a strong propensity of the voluminous and friable vegetations to embolize.

In fact, it is possible not to find a vegetation using echocardiography within the clinical profile of endocarditis accompanied by embolisms.

Obstructive vegetations

Vegetations of such large volume that they lead to obstruction of a valve orifice are rare, but are easily identifiable using echocardiography. This particular evolving form of vegetation, called 'obstructive', frequently has a fungal aetiology and traditionally affects the auriculoventricular valves.

Right-heart endocarditis

In the majority of cases the endocarditis is located in the left heart, and right-heart endocarditis is rare (5–10% of all cases of endocarditis). The vegetations generally affect healthy valves and may be observed:

- on pacing wires
- during the course of a contamination of a venous catheter
- in the context of highly virulent bacterial septicaemia
- in immunosuppressed patients
- in intravenous drug abuse
- in ventilated patients.

Most often, right-heart endocarditis is associated with a left location. It may complicate restrictive interventricular communication where the vegetations are located on the edges of the interventricular communication and the tricuspid valve or, less often the pulmonary valve.

Diagnostic pitfalls due to destructive lesions of endocarditis

These pitfalls most frequently relate to the TTE diagnosis of:

- endocardial abscesses
- ruptured chordae (see page 62)
- valvular perforations.

The use of TEE is extremely valuable in these situations, as it can provide a complete survey of the different lesions.

Pitfalls when diagnosing abscesses

Abscesses are found in 20–30% of cases of infective endocarditis. The advantage of echocardiography (TTE and/or TEE) resides in its detection and surveillance of annular abscesses, the presence of which indicates a major evolving complication. However, in spite of this performance, diagnosis of abscesses is still sometimes difficult in the situations described below.

Atypical morphological appearance of the abscess

Typically, an annular abscess appears in 2D echocardiography as a more or less rounded, encapsulated chamber that is devoid of echo; it is perivalvular, developed in contact with the annulus, and is sometimes moved by a systolic expansion (expansive anechoic neochamber) (Fig. 6.39).

The commonest site for abscessed lesions is the aortic annulus. Other echocardiographic appearances, less suggestive of abscess, are possible. They reflect the three developmental phases of the abscess (Fig. 6.40):

- Presuppurative phase: a hyperechoic abnormal para-annular thickening (> 10 mm) is observed at an early stage of abscess formation, before necrosis occurs.

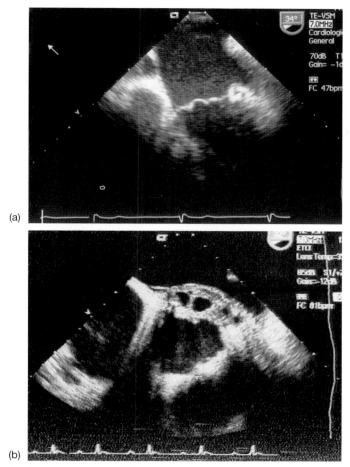

Figure 6.39   Abscesses viewed in TEE: (a) small 'cyst-like' abscesses of the mitral annulus; (b) abscess of the posterior aortic annulus in the form of two neochambers.

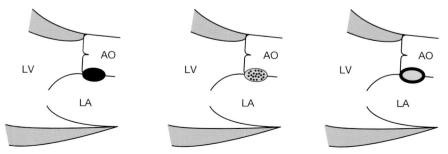

Figure 6.40   The three stages of development of an abscess of the aortomitral triangle (see text). AO, aorta; LA, left atrium; LV, left ventricle.

- Suppurative phase: a mass of abnormal heterogeneous echoes is seen due to the presence of necrotic material inside the abscess.
- Prefistulation stage: an encapsulated chamber with a thick shell corresponding to an evolving stage of the abscess, which often precedes fistulation.

These particular appearances only achieve their full value when considered together with the clinical context and the evolution of the echocardiographic images.

Small volume of the abscess
The size of abscesses varies from several millimetres to several centimetres. Echocardiography may be caught out in the case of small abscesses (> 5 mm), especially incipient abscesses, or periprosthetic abscesses (Box 6.12).

For small aortic abscesses, the diagnostic sensitivity of TTE is mediocre when the aortic walls are atheromatous or calcified. TEE is markedly superior to TTE in detecting abscesses of small volume.

Atypical location of annular abscesses
Abscesses are generally found at the level of the aortomitral fibrous triangle, at the junction between the posterior sinus of Valsalva and the base of the large mitral valve (posterior aortic para-annular abscess).

Other locations are possible, particularly for smaller abscesses, which makes them more difficult to detect. These locations are responsible for false-negative results (see Box 6.12). For example, small abscesses involving the connection between the interventricular septum is and the aortic annulus, which may develop into a ventricular septal defect. Likewise, small paravalvular mitral abscesses still frequently go undiagnosed.

Mistaken diagnosis of annular abscesses
The causes of false-positive results are summarized in Box 6.13. They are generally due to endocarditis on aortic prostheses (valvular or vascular).

Variable anatomical extent of abscesses
Abscesses of the aortic annulus may be highly localized or even circumferential, thereby destroying the whole of the fibrous annulus and leading to an aorto-ventricular dislocation. The operator should be aware during the echocardiographic examination of this particular anatomical shape of abscess. Finally, multiple abscesses of the aortic annulus may lead to genuine destruction of tissue.

Fistulation of abscesses in an adjacent structure
Fistulation of abscesses may occur in the aorta, LV, right chambers or the pericardium. It is vital to be able to recognize fistulation early, due to the major risks of infection and haemodynamic consequences.

However, fistulations may escape detection on TTE, although TEE has major advantages in their diagnosis. TEE enables visualization of even the small pinholes of a fistulated abscess. 2D colour Doppler allows detection of the abscessed pocket communicating with the aorta due to an abnormal diastolic filling flow,

Box 6.12   Causes of false-negative results relating to abscesses

- Incipient abscesses
- Anterior aortic para-annular abscesses
- Small mitral paravalvular abscesses
- Tricuspid or pulmonary annular abscesses
- Multiple abscesses of the aortic annulus
- Paraprosthetic abscesses masked by the valve prosthesis (screening effect)
- Massive calcifications of the aortic annulus leading to a 'masking effect'

in the case of fistulation in the ascending aorta. Fistulation of an abscess of the aortomitral triangle in the outflow chamber of the LV is indicated by an abnormal systolic filling flow. Finally, a major risk is represented by the rupture of an abscess in the free pericardium, which may lead to cardiac tamponade.

Pitfalls when diagnosing valvular perforations

The value of TEE in detecting valvular perforations is well documented. Nevertheless, it should be noted that there are diagnostic difficulties when using TEE when the perforation:

- is small in size (< 5 mm)
- affects the aortic valve (the diagnosis of mitral perforation is easier)
- is not located in the main valve body but is close to the coaptation zone of the valves
- is multiple.

Box 6.13   Causes of false-positive results relating to abscesses in endocarditis

- Aortic para-annular calcifications
- Periprosthetic annular fibrous formation
- Periprosthetic encapsulated haematoma
- Haematoma of the native aorta in the process of organization
- False aortic aneurysm following a Bentall surgical procedure
- False aneurysm of the aortomitral triangle
- Aneurysm of the sinus of Valsalva
- Collection of liquid in the transverse Theile sinus

PITFALLS WHEN QUANTIFYING VALVULAR REGURGITATION

Doppler echocardiography has become the method of choice for quantifying valvular regurgitation, slowly replacing angiography.

The echocardiographic evaluation of the importance of a valvular leak is based on:

- a study of the haemodynamic consequences of the leak
- a Doppler analysis of the regurgitant flow.

When faced with valvular regurgitation, the operator must work through all the phases of the echocardiographic examination (M-mode, 2D imaging, spectral and colour Doppler) in order to provide and compare with one another the maximum possibe number of measured parameters. These quantitative parameters, collected transthoracically and/or transoesophageally, are numerous, as no single parameter in itself provides sufficient information. Knowledge of the limitations specific to each parameter is required. Despite the good development of echocardiographic techniques, quantification of a valvular leak remains somewhat imperfect, due to the multiplicity of factors that can influence the different parameters involved. The echocardiographic pitfalls relating to the measurement and interpretation of these parameters are discussed for MR and AR conjointly.

PITFALLS WHEN EVALUATING THE HAEMODYNAMIC CONSEQUENCES OF A VALVULAR LEAK

The size of a mitral or aortic valvular leak may be assessed in an approximate manner by means of:

- the degree of dilatation of the LV (MR and AR) and the left atrium (MR)
- the existence of pulmonary arterial hypertension (MR) (see page 199).

However, the dilatation of the left chambers is an unreliable measure, and depends as much on the age of the leak as it does on its size. Typically, a large, chronic valvular leak carries an increased volume of flow from the LV, which becomes dilated and hyperkinetic. This left ventricular dilatation is usually greater in chronic AR than in chronic MR. Interpretation remains difficult in the case of severe dysfunction of the LV, and this is often responsible for an underestimation of the mitral leak. Dilatation of the LV may be absent in acute valvular leaks, where only hyperkinesia is present. Moreover, many smaller leaks do not show up echocardiographically, as the dimensions of the left chambers remain within normal limits.

In fact, dilatation of the left atrium is often multifactorial and depends, of course, on the degree and age of the MR, but also on the presence of a continuous arrhythmia through atrial fibrillation or an associated arterial hypertension. It is difficult, therefore, to predict the degree of MR based on this criterion alone. However, the observation of pulmonary hypertension is a solid argument in favour of the extensive nature of the MR when there is no other cause. Nevertheless, the influence of the size and compliance of the left atrium on the increase in pulmonary pressures must be taken into account:

- pulmonary hypertension may be only moderate in cases of moderate but longstanding MR with marked dilatation of the left atrium
- pulmonary hypertension is generally severe in cases of acute MR involving a small, non-compliant left atrium.

Pitfalls of Doppler analysis of a valvular leak

Cardiac Doppler has taken a paramount position in the quantification of valvular regurgitations. Several Doppler parameters for assessing the size of a valvular leak have been proposed (Box 6.14). The multiplicity of these parameters reflects the absence of an ideal reference method. The quantification of a valvular leak therefore rests on a set of parameters collected during the echo Doppler examination. This set of data enables the classification of valvular leaks into four grades – minimal (1/4), moderate (2/4), medium (3/4) and large (4/4) – with a certain amount of overlap possible between the different echocardiographic grades.

However, there are numerous technical pitfalls and diagnostic limitations to be aware of when using Doppler parameters. Firstly, it must be emphasized that the measurement of the maximum velocity of the MR (often exceeding 4 m/s) obtained using continuous Doppler does not allow quantification of the MR. In fact, the maximum velocity depends, above all, on the left intraventricular systolic pressures. It is lower in the case of low pressures (e.g. a drop in blood pressure) and higher (6–8 m/s) in the case of intraventricular hyperpressure (AS, hypertrophic cardiomyopathy). Other pitfalls of Doppler echocardiography con-

---

Box 6.14   Doppler parameters used to quantify a valvular leak

- The acoustic intensity and image density of the Doppler signal
- The duration of the turbulence during systole (MR) or diastole (AR)
- The increase in the maximum velocity of the anteroretrograde flow (in the absence of an associated valvular stenosis)
- The extent and size of the regurgitant jet
- The diameter of the regurgitant jet at its origin (vena contracta)
- The regurgitation fraction
- The ratio of the velocity–time integrals (MR)
- The degree of pulmonary hypertension (AR)
- The subisthmic end-diastolic velocity (AR)
- The appearance of the pulmonary venous flow (MR)
- The indices of the PISA method

AR, atrial regurgitation; MR, mitral regurgitation; PISA, proximal isovelocity surface area.

cern the parameters described below, which are used in the quantification of a valvular leak.

2D colour Doppler study of the extent and size of the regurgitant jet

2D colour Doppler is still the most popular and most widely used method, although its limitations are many. The limitations of this method are linked to the multiple, often uncontrollable, factors that determine the extent and size of the regurgitant jet (Box 6.15). Important among these factors is the direction of the jet, as the degree of the leak will be underestimated if the jet is eccentric or adherent to neighbouring structures (Fig. 6.41). In particular, when using 2D colour Doppler there is at risk of underestimating the degree of an eccentric MR adhering to the walls of the left atrium, due to the prolapse of a mitral valve or to ruptured mitral chordae. Likewise, paraprosthetic regurgitations may also transform into adherent jets, which will lead to an underestimation of the leak. This particular adherence of jets to cardiac walls is explained by the Coanda effect: the jet studied in a plane perpendicular to the wall spreads across its surface and remains relatively narrow.

The quantitative analysis of a valvular leak is also hampered by the presence of multiple jets in colour Doppler, where it is difficult to draw conclusions regarding the severity of the leak.

In order to appreciate the importance of the MR, the maximum and relative surface areas of the regurgitant jet (surface area of the jet/surface area of the LA)

Box 6.15   Factors determining the extent and size of the regurgitant jet

- The importance and the kinetic energy of the leak
- The size of the regurgitant orifice
- The size and compliance of the receiving chamber
- The load conditions (preload or afterload)
- The period of the cardiac cycle under consideration
- The direction of the regurgitant jet (central or eccentric jet)
- The temporal variations of the regurgitation
- The 'free' or adherent nature of the jet
- The number of regurgitant jets
- Technical factors: patient echogenicity, spatial resolution of the echocardiogram, level of colour gains and filters, image frequency, emission frequency, size of colour sector, post-treatment of the image, etc.
- The echocardiographic projections studied
- The echocardiographic route used: transthoracic or transoesophageal (monoplanar or multiplanar)
- The experience of the examiner

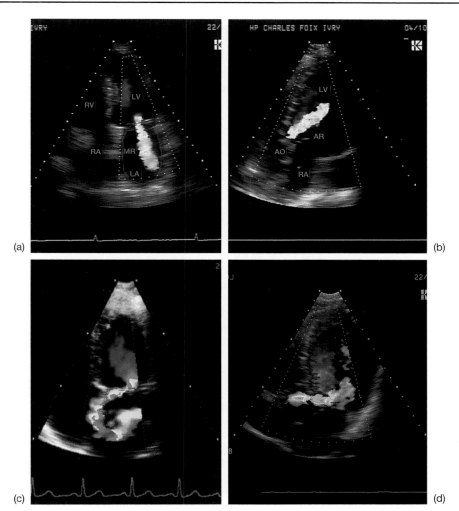

Figure 6.41   Valvular leaks explored in transthoracic 2D colour Doppler: (a) central, moderate mitral regurgitation (MR) (surface area MR/surface area LA = 32%); (b) central aortic regurgitation (AR); (c) eccentric major MR, with the jet directed towards the interatrial septum; (d) eccentric AR directed towards the mitral valve. AO, aorta; LA, left atrium; LV, left ventricle; RA, right atrium; RV, right ventricle.

are often measured using planimetry in 2D Doppler. In fact, the surface area of the MR determined using colour Doppler depends, of course, on the severity of the regurgitation, but also on many other factors, such as the haemodynamic status of the patient or the gain levels used in the recording. The higher the colour gain, the larger the leak appears on the screen. Moreover, the inter- and intraobserver variability in measuring the surface area of the regurgitated jet in colour Doppler is significant, varying by 15–20%. The threshold values of the jet surface area suggesting a large MR are 8 cm² (TTE) and 6 cm² (TEE). Finally, an underestimation of the MR is more frequent in cases of significant dilatation of the LA, in both TTE and TEE.

In practice, the analysis of the MR or AR jet using 2D colour Doppler usually makes it possible to distinguish between minimal leaks (grade 1) and major leaks (grade 4). The problem of quantification most often concerns intermediate sized leaks (grades 2 and 3).

Measuring the diameter of the regurgitant jet at its origin (vena contracta)

The measurement of the width of the jet at its origin allows a good evaluation of the size of the valvular leak. The measurement should be made using colour Doppler at the level of the narrowest part of the regurgitant jet through the valvular orifice corresponding to the vena contracta (Fig. 6.42). It may be carried out using TTE or, preferably, TEE (Fig. 6.43).

The advantage of measuring the width of the jet at the vena contracta is that it is less dependent on the haemodynamic conditions and, in particular, on the afterload, than it is on the regurgitation fraction. The limitations of this method are linked to the factors that determine the width of the vena contracta (Box 6.16). In fact, the measurement of the diameter of a colour jet implicitly assumes that the regurgitant orifice is roughly circular. This is far from true in many cases, as there is a wide variety of orifice shapes, of which only one dimension is measured.

The presence of eccentric jets or non-circular regurgitant orifices makes application of the colour Doppler method difficult. In the case of an eccentric jet, a measurement carried out with precision in 2D colour Doppler may be adequate under certain circumstances. However, the method is unusable in the case of multiple regurgitant jets. In practice, the diameter of the regurgitant jet should be measured strictly at its origin. Beyond this point the jet widens rapidly, which can lead to significant variation in the diameter over just a few

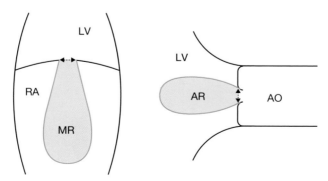

Figure 6.42 Measurement of the diameter of mitra regurgitation (MR) and aortic regurgitation (AR) jets at their origin (vena contracta) using 2D colour Doppler TTE. AO, aorta; RA, right atrium; LV, left ventricle.

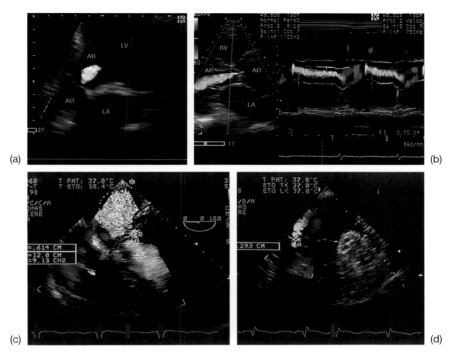

(a)

(b)

(c)

(d)

Figure 6.43 Quantification of valvular leaks measuring the vena contracta (VC) in colour Doppler TTE (a, b) and colour Doppler TEE (c, d). (a) Moderate aortic regurgitation (AR) with VC = 2.6 mm in 2D; (b) medium AR with VC = 7 mm in colour M-mode; (c) major MR with surface area = 9.1 cm^2, VC = 6.1 mm; (d) moderate to medium eccentric mitral regurgitation (MR) with VC = 2.9 mm in this projection.

Box 6.16   Factors determining the width of the vena contracta

- The visualization of the vena contracta: integral or incomplete?

- The measurement angle in relation to the axis of the regurgitant jet (risk of overestimation of the vena contracta if the angle is oblique)

- The nature of the regurgitant jet: central or eccentric (oblique) jet

- The shape of the regurgitant orifice: circular or non-circular

- The number of regurgitant jets: single or multiple

- A bicuspid aortic valve (asymmetric valves)

- Aortic subvalvular membranous stenosis

- Insufficient adjustment of the colour gains

- An acoustic shadow cast over the vena contracta by valvular calcification

- The recording route: transthoracic or transoesophageal

- The mode of colour Doppler measurement: 2D or M-mode

millimetres. The measurement is best made using 2D colour Doppler (MR and AR). In colour M-mode, the measurement should be made as close as possible to the aortic cusps (AR). The adjustment of the colour gains is also important: overly high gains will overestimate the diameter of the jet and, therefore, the size of the leak; gains that are set too low may lead to an underestimate of the leak. It is necessary in all cases to use the zoom and to take the mean value of several measurements. A length of the vena contracta of > 6 mm corresponds to a significant mitral or aortic leak. Some studies propose threshold values of 5–6.5 mm. In fact, the threshold values depend on the spatial resolution used during the colour Doppler imaging. Finally, there are overlap zones between leak grades 2 and 3, making the differentiation between these two grades difficult when using the length of the vena contracta as the sole criterion.

Calculation of the regurgitation fraction

In theory, calculation of the regurgitation fraction (RF) is the most precise method of quantifying a valvular leak. The calculation consists of comparing the mitral output (O_M) and the aortic output (O_A) calculated using pulsed echo Doppler:

$$RF = \frac{O_M - O_A}{O_M} \text{ (for MR)}$$

$$RF = \frac{O_A - O_M}{O_A} \text{ (for AR)}$$

An RF value of > 50% suggests a significant leak (grades 3 to 4).

However, this quantitative method may be somewhat time consuming for routine use, requiring meticulous measurements that are sometimes difficult to reproduce. The limitations of the method are also numerous (Box 6.17). The imprecision in the echocardiographic measurement of the mitral and aortic surface areas is the principal limitation to calculating the RF using echo Doppler. Errors can also occur in the measurement of the annular diameters and/or the VTIs. Moreover, this method is no longer valid if AR, or MS associated with the MR, is present. In the case of AR, the method is usable in the absence of AS or MR, but the method is difficult to apply in cases of atrial fibrillation or in

---

Box 6.17   Limitations of the calculation of the regurgitation fraction using the aortic and mitral outputs

- Any error in the measurement of the annular diameters is squared
- The aortic orifice is circular in shape, the mitral orifice is elliptical
- The variations in the calibre of the mitral orifice are low during systole; those of the mitral orifice are constant throughout diastole
- The method is not applicable if there is an associated valvulopathy
- Atrial fibrillation leads to variable velocity–time integrals
- The reproducibility of measurements of the atrial and mitral outputs is moderate

carriers of a valve prosthesis. However, the method gives good results when it is used in suitably selected patients.

The complexity of the calculation of the RF in the case of MR led to proposals for the use of the simple ratio of the VTIs of the mitral flow and the aortic flow. A ratio of > 1.3 corresponds to an RF of > 40%. However, this method too is valid ony in the absence of MS or AR.

Measurement of the pressure half-time of aortic regurgitation

This pressure half-time (PHT) of aortic regurgitation ($T_{\frac{1}{2}p}$) is measured using the AR flow recorded in continuous Doppler (Fig. 6.44). The shorter the PHT, the more severe the AR. A PHT of < 300 ms suggests significant AR.

The factors determining the length of the PHT of the AR are summarized in Box 6.18. These factors are technical or haemodynamic in origin, and familiarity with them is necessary in order to avoid incorrect results (Figs 6.45 and 6.46).

In practice, measurement of the PHT requires excellent definition of the contours of the AR spectrum, recorded in its totality with the early diastolic velocity exceeding 3 m/s. However, it is frequently found that, for eccentric leaks, beam alignment in continuous Doppler is extremely difficult, which renders the measurement of the PHT highly unpredictable. Moreover, any increase in the end-diastolic pressure of the LV decreases the PHT, which leads to a risk of overestimating the AR. Finally, the PHT is markedly shortened (< 200 ms) in cases of acute AR, due to a sharp rise in the end-diastolic pressure of the LV (see Box 6.23 and Fig. 6.52).

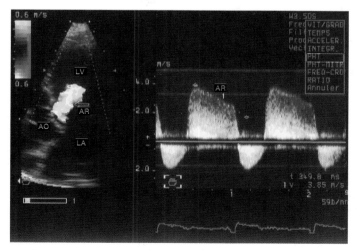

Figure 6.44 Correct recording of aortic regurgitation (AR) in continuous Doppler coupled with 2D colour imaging (good alignment). Perfect definition of the contours of the AR spectrum (early diastolic velocity = 3.8 m/s; $T_{\frac{1}{2}p}$ = 349 ms). AO, aorta; LA, left atrium; LV, left ventricle.

> **Box 6.18   Factors determining the duration of the pressure half-time ($T_{\frac{1}{2}p}$) in aortic regurgitation**
>
> **Technical factors**
> - The degree of alignment over the regurgitant jet
> - The integrity of the aortic regurgitant envelope
> - The definition of the spectral envelope
>
> **Haemodynamic factors**
> - The end-diastolic pressure of the left ventricle (decreased $T_{\frac{1}{2}p}$ indicates associated aortic stenosis, ischaemic or hypertrophic cardiac pathology, cardiac insufficiency)
> - The degree of change in the diastolic function of the left ventricle (decreased $T_{\frac{1}{2}p}$ indicates a disturbance of left ventricular compliance)
> - An acute aortic regurgitation ($T_{\frac{1}{2}p} < 200$ ms)
> - The systolic arterial resistance
> - The aortic compliance

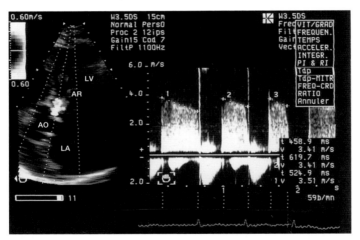

Figure 6.45   Variability in the pressure half-time of aortic regurgitation (AR) (524, 619 and 458 ms) where there is continuous arrhythmia due to atrial fibrillation. AO, aorta; LA, left atrium; LV, left ventricle.

Measurement of the subisthmic end-diastolic velocity of aortic regurgitation

A positive diastolic regurgitant jet recorded using pulsed Doppler in the ascending aorta reflects the size of the aortic leak. An end-diastolic velocity of > 0.2 m/s suggests a major AR. The measurement of the end-diastolic regurgitant jet remains valid in the presence of an associated AS. The limitations of this method are predominantly technical in nature, or are due to associated pathologies disrupting the measurement (Box 6.19). In certain cases, principally older

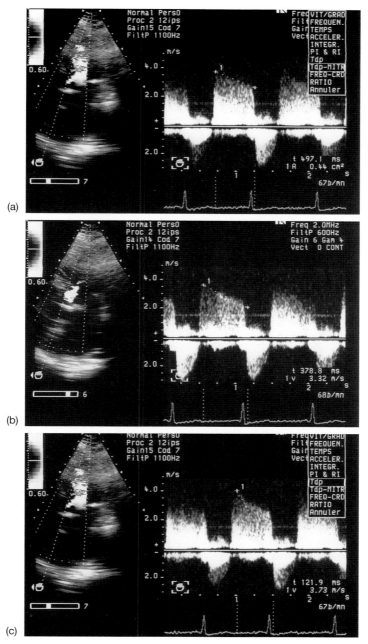

(a)

(b)

(c)

Figure 6.46 Variability in the pressure half-time of aortic regurgitation (497 and 378 ms) as a function of the Doppler projection and the definition of the diastolic slope. All measured in the same patient.

Box 6.19   Factors determining the subisthmic end-diastolic velocity of the aortic regurgitation

- Technical factors:
  - degree of alignment over the regurgitant jet
  - definition of the spectrum in end-diastole
  - correct recording site (downstream of the left subclavicular artery)

- Associated pathologies:
  - aortic coarctation
  - arterial canal
  - aortic dissection
  - aortopulmonary fistula

- Heart rate:
  - tachycardia (> 120 beats/minute)
  - bradycardia (< 50 beats/minute)

- Aortic compliance

- Acute aortic regurgitation

subjects, the aortic arch may be difficult to pick up. In terms of adjusting the machine controls, it is vital to reduce the wall filters to a minimum in order to visualize correctly an end-diastolic regurgitant jet. Extreme variations in heart rate can also influence the measurement of the end-diastolic velocity of the AR. The size of the diastolic regurgitant jet also depends on the aortic compliance, which is often low in older subjects. Finally, acute AR leads to annulment of the subisthmic end-diastolic velocity (see Box 6.23).

Appearance of the pulmonary venous flow

The analysis of the pulmonary venous flow (PVF) using pulsed Doppler is useful for the quantification of mitral regurgitation.

Normal PVF comprises two positive waves, systolic and diastolic, and a retrograde wave linked to the atrial contraction (see Fig. 9.8, page 172).

In the presence of a major MR, an end-systolic or holosystolic inversion of the PVF is encountered. Significant MR can be practically ruled out when the velocity of the systolic wave is greater than that of the diastolic wave. In fact, severe MR involves an inverted flow in 93% of cases. However, this systolic inversion of the PVF depends on several factors (Box 6.20). The diagnostic pitfalls principally relate to eccentric MR flows through a prolapse of the mitral valve. The direction of the regurgitant jet, as determined from the shape of the MVP, influences the PVF in the following manner (Fig. 6.47):

- prolapse of the large mitral valve generates a jet adhering to the lateral wall of the left atrium, and a systolic inversion preferentially involves the flow in the left pulmonic veins
- prolapse of the small mitral valve is responsible for a jet directed towards the interatrial septum and for a preferential regurgitant jet in the right pulmonic veins.

Box 6.20   Factors determining the systolic inversion of the pulmonary venous flow in the case of mitral regurgitation

- The size of the mitral leak
- The direction of the regurgitant jet
- The size of the left atrium
- The left atrial compliance
- Associated anomalies (atrial fibrillation, mitral stenosis, left ventricular dysfunction)

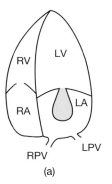
(a)

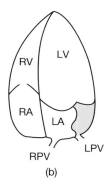
(b)

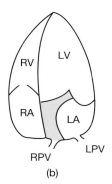
(b)

Figure 6.47   Trajectories of the mitral regurgitation (MR) jet according to the MR mechanism. (a) Central MR due   to annular dilatation; (b) eccentric MR due to prolapse of the large mitral valve; (c) eccentric MR due to prolapse of the small mitral valve. LA, left atrium; LPV, left pulmonic vein; LV, left ventricle; RA, right atrium; RPV, right pulmonic vein; RV, right ventricle.

It is therefore necessary to search systematically for the systolic flow reversal at the level of the right and left pulmonic veins, due to the possibility of an elective inversion in one of the four pulmonic veins. This search involves the use of TEE, with which it is possible to visualize the four veins. In TTE, only the upper right pulmonic vein is generally accessible.

The size and compliance of the left atrium also influence the PVF in cases of MR. The systolic inversion of the flow is all the freer if the left atrium is smaller and less compliant. In fact, moderate MR is associated with a normal PVF, or only a reduced systolic wave. However, the reduction of the systolic wave of the PVF may also be seen in other circumstances, such as in continuous arrhythmia due to atrial fibrillation, an MS or severe left ventricular dysfunction. Only the systolic inversion of the PVF constitutes a reliable and specific sign of major MR.

Study of the convergence zone
During the course of valvular regurgitation the convergence zone centred on the leaking orifice can be visualized using 2D colour Doppler. This hemispherical convergence zone corresponds to the constant-velocity laminar flow that

converges on the regurgitating orifice. This flow is identifiable in colour Doppler by modifying the aliasing level on the velocity scale (Figs 6.48 and 6.49). The convergence zone or PISA (proximal isovelocity surface area) serves as a means of quantifying a valvular leak. According to the principle of output continuity, the output calculated at the level of the convergence zone is equal to the output of the regurgitating orifice.

In practice, the distance separating the regurgitating orifice from the first aliasing (which corresponds to the radius (r) of the convergence zone), the velocity of which is known (aliasing velocity), is measured. Therefore, knowing the value of r, it is possible to calculate the surface area of the convergence zone using the formula $2\pi r^2$. The measurement of r should be done particularly carefully, as any error is squared in the calculation of the surface area.

The other indices allowing for the quantification of MR or AR can then be calculated, such as:

- the instantaneous maximum regurgitated output: RO = $2\pi r^2 V$
- the regurgitant orifice area: ROA = RO/V_{max} of the MR (or of the AR)
- regurgitated volume per cardiac cycle: V_R = ROA × VTI of the MR (or of the AR).

In practice, use of the PISA method requires rigorous technique. Failure to observe the necessary conditions for examinations (Box 6.21) may lead to incorrect results. Likewise, it is necessary to understand the limitations of the method in order to avoid misleading results (Box 6.22).

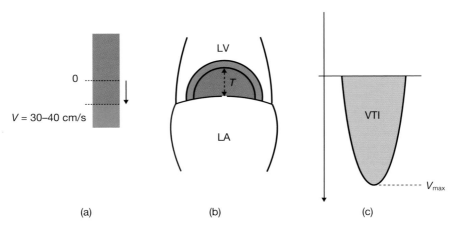

Figure 6.48 Examination technique for the convergence zone of an mitral regurgitation (MR) according to the PISA method. (a) The zero line of the velocity (V) scale is moved downward (aliasing level 30–40 cm/s). (b) Detection and measurement of the radius of the intra-left ventricular convergence zone. (c) Collection of the MR spectrum in continuous Doppler, which enables the measurement of the velocity–time integral (VTI) and the maximum velocity (V_{max}). LA, left atrium; LV, left ventricle.

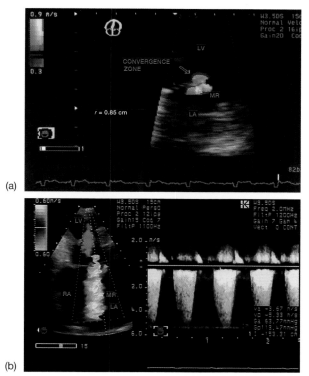

(a)

(b)

Figure 6.49   Quantification of the mitral regurgitation (MR) by means of the PISA method (TTE). (a) Study of the convergence zone: radius (r) = 0.85 cm, aliasing velocity (V) = 30 cm/s. (b) MR recorded using colour and continuous Doppler: maximum velocity (Vmax) = 533 cm/s, velocity–time integral (VTI) = 153 cm. regurgitated output (RO) = (2 × 3.14 × 0.852 × 30) = 135 ml/s; regurgitant orifice area (ROA) = 135/533 = 0.25 cm2; regurgitant volume (VR) = 0.25 × 153 = 38.2 ml. In summary, the MR is of medium size (grade 3/4).LA, left atrium; LV, left ventricle; RA, right atrium.

The limitations of the PISA method are principally linked to:

- poor examination conditions, not allowing for perfect visualization of the convergence zone or the precise measurement of its radius
- a possible deformation of the convergence zone
- the variations in the radius of the convergence zone over the course of the cardiac cycle
- an inappropriate selection of the aliasing velocity.

Deformation of the convergence zone

The PISA method assumes that the convergence zone, situated just upstream of the regurgitant orifice, is hemispherical. However, its shape is only hemispherical if the regurgitant orifice is circular and located within a plane. In reality, the convergence zone may be 'deformed' in certain situations.

The principal causes of deformation of the convergence zone are:

- certain aetiologies of valvular insufficiencies (MVP, bicuspid aortic valve, annular ectasia of the aorta, aneurysm of the ascending aorta, etc.)
- a complex, non-circular geometry of the mitral or aortic orifice
- an incorrectly adjusted aliasing level
- a confinement phenomenon.

These factors result, in particular, to non-hemispherical shapes of the convergence zone, such as:

- A truncated or semi-elliptical hemisphere, which is observed in certain MRs due to MVP. These shapes lead to an overestimation of the valvular leak.

Box 6.21   Conditions for examining the convergence zone of a valvular leak when using 2D colour Doppler

- Apical cross-section of the four chambers (mitral regurgitation (MR)) or of the two left chambers with the aorta (aortic regurgitation (AR))
- Reduced coloured sector (30°)
- Green range (turbulence) removed
- Zero line moved downwards (MR) or upwards (AR)
- Colour gain correctly adjusted
- Image zoomed
- Convergence zone detected in cine mode
- Radius (r) of the convergence zone measured precisely
- Aliasing velocity (V) supplied by the apparatus transferred to the calculating software

---

Box 6.22   Potential limitations of the PISA method

Convergence zone
- Poorly visualized: patient hypoechogenicity; sensitivity of colour Doppler (image frequencies, emission frequency, etc.), adjustment of colour gains
- Deformed (non-hemispherical): truncated hemisphere, hemi-ellipse, 'larger' than a hemisphere

Radius of convergence zone
- Poorly measured: patients with low echogenicity, poor definition of the plane of the valve annulus
- Variable over the course of the cardiac cycle
- Difficult to measure when a tiny leak is present

Aliasing velocity
- Too high: 'flattened' convergence zone
- Too low: 'enlarged' convergence zone

- An 'enlarged' hemisphere (> 180°), as observed in cases of annular ectasia of the aorta, where the valves have the appearance of an inverted funnel (Fig. 6.50). This shape leads to a risk of underestimating the size of the leak (Fig. 6.51).

In both situations it is necessary to make an angular correction by multiplying the regurgitated output by the ratio of the angle $\alpha/180$ (RO = $2\pi r^2 V \alpha/180$). The angle α, which is the angle delimited by the valves, in fact corresponds to the angle of the convergence zone.

Finally, if there is strong compression of the convergence zone by the ventricular walls (confinement phenomenon), the PISA method should be abandoned.

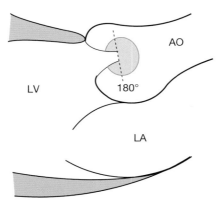

Figure 6.50   Study of the convergence zone of AR in the case of aneurysmal dilatation of the initial aorta. In this case, the convergence zone is larger than a hemisphere and the angle α is > 180°. AO, aorta; LA, left atrium; LV, left ventricle.

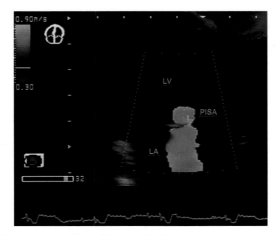

Figure 6.51   Particular shape of the left intraventricular convergence zone: an 'enlarged' hemisphere. LA, left atrium; LV, left ventricle; PISA, proximal isovelocity surface area.

This situation occurs principally in certain lateralized MRs of prolapses of the small mitral valve, but also in certain restrictive MRs.

Variations in the radius of the convergence zone
The radius of the convergence zone measured at a given moment corresponds to a maximum distance and does not account for the variations that may occur throughout the cardiac cycle. This is the case in MVPs, where an increase in the radius is generally observed in mid- to end-systole. In rheumatic MR, the radius of the convergence zone remains stable throughout systole. In functional MR, the radius often increases during early and end-systole. In fact, the variations in the radius of the convergence zone, which are clearly visible in colour M-mode, correspond to variations in the regurgitated output. In these situations the use of a mean value of radius is usually required.

Aliasing level
The convergence zone corresponds to the velocity of the first aliasing chosen by the operator in order to optimize the visualization of the zone. Most frequently, velocities of 30–40 cm/s of the aliasing zone are used, lowering the zero line of the velocity scale in cases of MR and raising it in cases of AR.

Choosing the optimum aliasing velocity is of paramount importance in order to quantify a valvular leak reliably. In fact, too high an aliasing velocity leads to a flattening of the convergence zone, and therefore to an underestimate of the regurgitated output. In contrast, too low a velocity leads to enlargement of the convergence zone, which results in an overestimation of the regurgitated output.

In spite of all these limitations, it is worth studying the convergence zone when quantifying valvular leaks. The criteria for a major MR or AR, established on the basis of the PISA method, are summarized in Table 6.7.

SPECIFIC CLINICAL SCENARIOS

It is necessary to set apart acute ARs and diastolic MRs that arise in a particular clinical context. Lack of familiarity with the echocardiographic indicators of these particular valvulopathies may lead to incorrect diagnoses. So-called 'dynamic MR' may be demonstrated using exercise echocardiography.

Acute aortic regurgitation (Fig. 6.52)
Acute AR may be secondary to an endocarditis, an aortic dissection or a valvular rupture of traumatic origin. In Doppler echocardiography, the consequences of a sharp elevation in the end-diastolic pressure of the LV, surpassing that of the LA, can be observed (Box 6.23). The LV is generally hyperkinetic and of normal dimensions.

Diastolic mitral regurgitation
Diastolic MR corresponds to a back flow of blood through the mitral orifice before the start of the contraction of the LV. The condition may exist in isolation or be associated with a systolic MR (Figs 6.52 and 6.53).

Table 6.7 Principal echo Doppler criteria for significant mitral regurgitation (MR) and and significant aortic regurgitation (AR)

Parameter	MR	AR
Spatial extension	At the base of the LA	Beyond the mitral funnel
Regurgitant surface area	> 6 cm² (TTE) > 8 cm² (TEE)	
Vena contracta	> 6 mm	> 6 mm
Regurgitated fraction	> 50%	> 50%
Pressure half-time		< 300 ms
End-diastolic velocity		> 0.2 m/s
Pulmonary venous flow	Systolic regurgitant jet	
PISA indices	RO > 140 ml/s ROA > 30 mm² V_R > 60 ml	ROA > 25–30 mm² V_R > 50–60 ml

LA, left atrium; PISA, proximal isovelocity surface area; RO, regurgitated output; ROA, regurgitant orifice area; TEE, transoesophageal echocardiography; TTE, transthoracic echocardiography; V_R, regurgitant volume.

Box 6.23   Echo Doppler signals in acute aortic regurgitation

- Premature closing of the mitral valve
- Premature opening of the aortic cusps
- A pressure half-time ($T_{1/2\,p}$) value < 200 ms
- An annulment of the subisthmic end-diastolic velocity (zero velocity)
- A hypernormal mitral flow with an elevated E/A ratio and short mitral $T_{1/2\,p}$
- An end-diastolic mitral regurgitation (Doppler equivalent of premature mitral closing)

Diastolic MR is observed in the following situations:

- atrioventricular block
- acute AR
- certain cases of elevated left ventricular end-diastolic pressure
- certain cases of restrictive-type anomalies in left ventricular filling.

Pulsed and continuous cardiac Doppler make it possible to show these pathologies and to study precisely their chronology and velocity.

Dynamic mitral regurgitation

The dynamic nature of certain MRs, such as ischaemic insufficiencies, may be demonstrated using exercise echocardiography. During exercise, it is possible during the course of a single examination to search for a possible change in

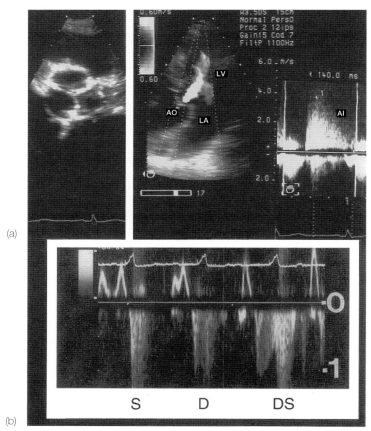

Figure 6.52 Particular valvular leaks. (a) Acute aortic regurgitation (AR) of endocardial origin. The pressure half-time ($T_{1/2 p}$) measured on the AR spectrum recorded in short continuous Doppler (140 ms). (b) Diastolic (D) mitral regurgitation (MR) recorded in a case of atrioventricular dissociation in a patient with a paceaker of the VVI mode. There is also mild systolic (S) MR. AO, aorta; DS, diastolic and systolic; LA, left atrium; LV, left ventricle. (Images by Dr T. Touche.)

the segmentary contractility and an evolution of the severity of the mitral leak. The leak may diminish during exercise, or, conversely, increase significantly. The detection of these dynamic mitral leaks is better during exercise than during stress echocardiography under Dobutamine. In fact, the test using Dobutamine reduces the severity of many dynamic leaks due to the fall in the afterload.

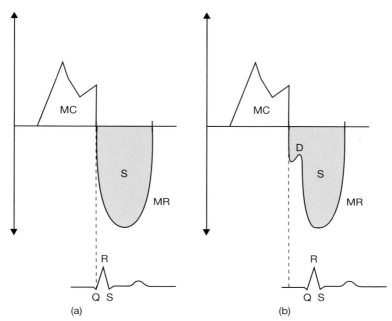

Figure 6.53 Mitral regurgitation (MR) recorded using continuous Doppler. (a) Systolic MR (S). (b) Diastolic MR (D) associated with a systolic MR (S); the vertical line indicates the beginning of the MR, which arises before the start of the QRS wave. MC, mitral closing.

7

Cardiac walls

The echocardiographic pitfalls relating to imaging of the cardiac walls are concerned with the diagnosis of:

- wall hypertrophy
- myocardial ischaemia
- pericardial lesions.

PITFALLS WHEN DIAGNOSING WALL HYPERTROPHY

In current practice, echocardiography is the method of choice for identifying and quantifying left ventricular hypertrophy (LVH). However, the method has certain limitations relating to:

- measuring the wall thicknesses
- calculating the myocardial mass of the left ventricle (LV)
- distinguishing between physiological and pathological LVH
- diagnosing primary hypertrophic cardiomyopathy.

The echocardiographic prevalence of LVH varies according to the population studied, the calculation method used and the criteria used to define it. LVH is present in about 35% of hypertensive patients. Echocardiography with Doppler tissue imaging (DTI) makes it possible to identify the early myocardial anomalies in hypertensive patients without ventricular hypertrophy. In fact, the diastolic myocardial velocities are significantly reduced in hypertensive patients compared with in normotensive patients, in the absence of LVH.

Pitfalls in measuring the wall thicknesses

M-mode measurements of the LV are vital in the diagnosis of left ventricular wall hypertrophy. The interpretation of the measured values (end-diastolic thickness of the septum and of the posterior wall of the LV) is only reliable if the strict quality criteria for M-mode recording are applied (Box 7.1). Conventionally, the M-mode examination is guided by the two-dimensional (2D) mode and begins in the left parasternal window. This makes it possible to obtain M-mode measurements of the base of the longitudinal cross-section. Other echocardiographic projections may be used (the short-axis parasternal view at the level of the papillary muscles below the mitral valve, or the subcostal view) if the parasternal long-axis view is not usable.

> **Box 7.1   Conditions for the echocardiographic measurement of left ventricular wall thicknesses**
>
> - Patient examined in left lateral decubitus position while resting
> - Transducer placed in the intercostal space, providing the best echocardiographic window
> - M-mode study carried out under 2D control (simultaneous 2D and M-mode views)
> - M-mode line placed at the papillary muscles–chordae junction, as identified in 2D
> - Examination depth of 17–21 cm in adults, selected according to heart size
> - Ideal M-mode paper speed 50 cm/s
> - Depth scale visible on the M-mode tracing
> - Real-time recording in M-mode over at least three cardiac cycles (average of the three interpretable measurements)
> - M-mode measurements made according to the convention chosen in advance

The causes of errors in the measurement of wall thicknesses are summarized in Box 7.2.

Poor definition of the endocardium

Poor echocardiographic definition of the endocardium may be due to an incorrect adjustment of the gain settings, in particular, or to the 'reject' or low echogenicity of the patient being examined.

In fact, the number of poorly echogenic patients is considerable, varying from 20% to 30% of cases, according to the recruitment factors used. Any echocardiographic measurement made in these patients should be treated with caution; such measurements may even be totally fallacious. Harmonic imaging techniques can be used to improve the definition of the ventricular walls in these particularly difficult patients.

> **Box 7.2   Causes of error in the M-mode measurement of wall thicknesses**
>
> - Poor echocardiographic definition of the wall endocardium
> - Imprecise identification of the end-diastole
> - Oblique M-mode angle in relation to the ventricular walls
> - Inclusion of the tricuspid apparatus, mitral chordae or false tendon in the measurement of the wall thicknesses
> - Presence of a subaortic septal rim or a muscular band
> - Presence of septal kinking

Imprecise detection of end-diastole

The detection of end-diastole affects the measurement of the wall thicknesses. End-diastole is identified according to the convention applied, whether this be the start of the Q wave of the QRS complex, or the peak of the R wave (Figs 7.1 and 7.2). Thus it is necessary to record the electrocardiogram (ECG) in parallel with the echocardiogram. This cannot be used when there is left bundle branch block.

Oblique M-mode angle in relation to the ventricular walls

If the M-mode angle is oblique in relation to the ventricular walls, the wall thicknesses will be overestimated (Fig. 7.3).

Normally, the M-mode line should be positioned perpendicular to the major or minor left ventricular axis and just below the free edge of the mitral valve. In

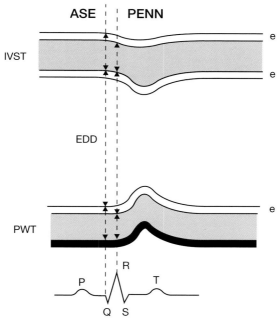

Figure 7.1   Two M-mode echocardiographic techniques for measuring the interventricular septal thickness (IVST), the ventricular end-diastolic diameter (EDD) and the posterior wall thickness (PWT) in end-diastole according to (Box 7.3):

- The American Society of Echocardiography (ASE) convention: at the beginning of the QRS complex, using the 'leading edge–leading edge' technique. The anterior endocardium (e) of the septum and of the posterior wall is included, and the posterior endocardium excluded, in the measurement of the wall thickness.
- The Pennsylvania (PENN) convention: at the peak of the R wave of the QRS complex, excluding the endocardium for the measurement of the wall thicknesses.

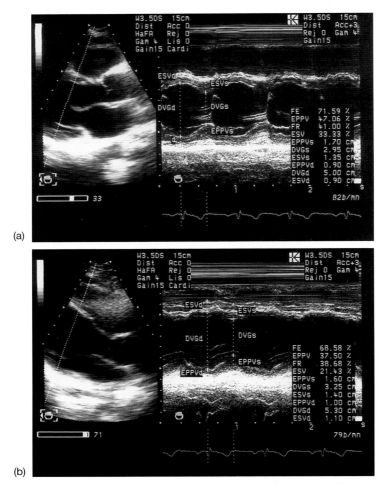

Figure 7.2 M-mode measurement of the wall thicknesses of the left ventricle. (a) Correct long-axis projection, perpendicular to the ventricular walls (interventricular septal thickness (IVST) = 9 mm, posterior wall thickness (PWT) = 9 mm). (b) Incorrect oblique projection overestimating the wall thickness (IVST = 11 mm, PWT = 10 mm) in the same patient.

practice, however, obtaining orthogonal cross-sections is sometimes difficult. In certain cases, this may be achieved by:

- positioning the ultrasound probe an intercostal space above, closer to the sternum, if the patient's echogenicity remains good
- making measurements in the subcostal window, if this is of good quality.

A new M-mode technique, called 'anatomical M-mode', is particularly useful in the case of oblique ventricular M-mode projections. It allows the overestimated M-mode measurements of the LV to be corrected (Fig. 7.4).

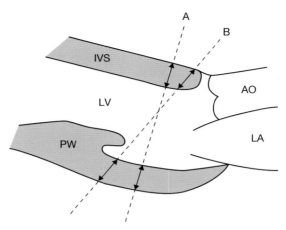

Figure 7.3 Measurements of the left ventricle (LV) during diastole in the parasternal, long-axis cross-section: (a) correct orthogonal M-mode projection; (b) oblique M-mode projection overestimating the wall thicknesses and the internal diameter of the LV. AO, aorta; IVS, interventricular septum; LA, left atrium; PW, posterior wall.

Box 7.3   The ASE and PENN formulae for calculating the left ventricular mass (LVM) based on the M-mode measurement of the diameter of the left ventricle (EDD), the interventricular septal thickness (IVST) and the posterior wall thickness (PWT) at end-diastole (see Fig. 7.1)

American Society of Echocardiography (ASE) formula:

$$LVM = 0.8[1.04 \times (EDD + IVST + PWT)^3 - EDD^3] + 0.6$$

Pennsylvania (PENN)/Devereux formula:

$$LVM = 1.04[(EDD + IVST + PWT)^3 - EDD^3] - 13.6$$

Inclusion of the tricuspid apparatus, mitral chordae or false septal tendon in the measurement of the wall thicknesses (Fig. 7.5)

When measuring the septum, care must be taken to distinguish between the tricuspid subvalvular apparatus and the anterior septal endocardial border. Between these two structures there is normally a clear, echo-free space. Likewise, the inclusion of the mitral chordae may lead to incorrect positioning of the measuring cursor when detecting the anterior border of the posterior wall of the LV. However, the M-mode slope of the posterior wall is greater than that of the chordae.

The presence of a false septal tendon may be responsible for an overestimation of the septal thickness. A false tendon, which is composed of muscular tissue, is transformed in 2D echocardiography into a linear structure attached to the left surface of the septum in the form of a bridge. It should be identified by careful echocardiographic examination of the septum in order to exclude it from the M-mode measurement of the septal thickness. In order to eliminate

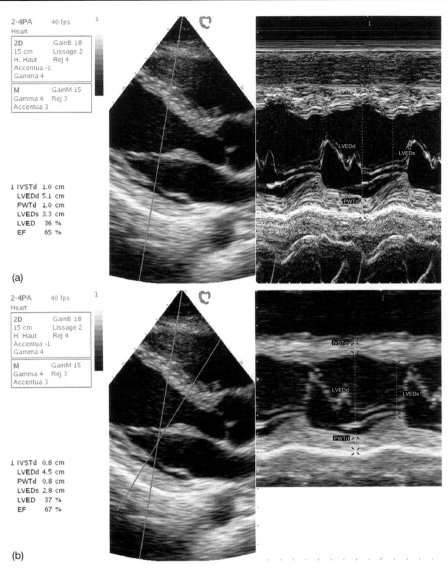

Figure 7.4 Anatomical M-mode echocardiographic technique (b) enabling the correction of the oblique measurement of the wall thicknesses of the left ventricle (a). IVSTd, interventricular septal thickness during diastole; LVEDd, left ventricular diameter during diastole; LVDs, left ventricular diameter during systole; PWTd, posterior wall thickness during diastole. (Imagic system, Kontron-Esaote.)

these anatomical sources of error, it is imperative to use multiple echocardiographic projections (lower left parasternal, minor axis, apical, subcostal) in order to obtain a clear, measurable and interpretable M-mode trace.

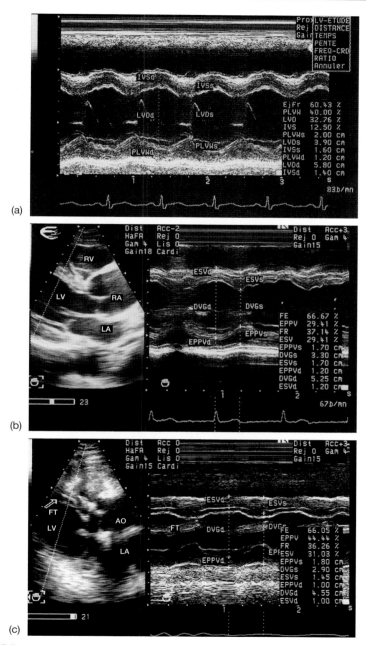

Figure 7.5 Anatomical causes of echocardiographic overestimation of the wall thicknesses. Possible mistaken inclusion in the M-mode measurement of (a) the tricuspid apparatus, (b) the mitral chordae or (c) the false septal tendon (FT). In these images, the measurements have been made correctly. AO, aorta; LA, left atrium; LV, left ventricle; RA, right atrium; RV, right ventricle.

Presence of a subaortic septal rim or a muscular band

The subaortic septal rim is defined as a hypertrophy located exclusively on the basal part of the interventricular septum, the diastolic thickness of which is > 13 mm. This rim is identifiable in the 2D parasternal, long-axis or apical cross-section (the two left chambers and the aorta). The rim may lead to an over-estimation of the septal thickness because of the use of an inappropriate M-mode projection. In order to avoid this pitfall, the M-mode line should be positioned below the septal rim (Figs 7.6 and 7.7). Use of the subcostal project-ion is sometimes preferred. A subaortic septal rim should be distinguished from a septal hypertrophy arising from hypertrophic obstructive cardiomyopathy (HOCM), which is an echocardiographic diagnostic pitfall to beware of (see Table 7.4).

Likewise, the presence of an abnormal muscular band of the right ventricle may obstruct the exact measurement of the septal thickness. The moderator band passes from the lower part of the interventricular septum to the anterior part of the right ventricle, where it is attached to the anterior papillary muscle. It may be identified by imaging multiple echocardiographic cross-sections of the right heart.

Presence of septal kinking (angulation)

Septal kinking is a particular morphology of the septum that is identifiable in the parasternal, long-axis cross-section (see Fig. 7.7). Normally, the angulation of the septum in relation to the axis of the aorta falls between 140° and 125°. In the case of septal kinking (aortoseptal angle ≤ 90°), a poorly directed ultra-sound beam approaches the septum obliquely, giving an appearance of false septal hypertrophy (Fig. 7.8).

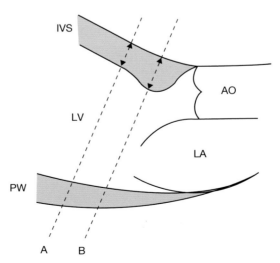

Figure 7.6   Subaortic septal rim: (a) optimum M-mode projection; (b) M-mode projection passing through the rim and overestimating the septal thickness. AO, aorta; IVS, interventricular septum; LA, left atrium; LV, left ventricle; PW, posterior wall.

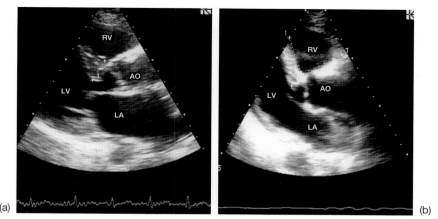

Figure 7.7   Anatomical causes of echocardiographic overestimation of the septal thickness: (a) subaortic septal rim; (b) septal kinking with an aortoseptal angle of 80°. AO, aorta; LA, left atrium; LV, left ventricle; RV, right ventricle.

Thus it is often the case that the probe has to be repositioned in order to avoid the septal kinking that may lead to overestimation of the thickness of the septum. As far as possible, the M-mode line should be perpendicular to the septum and the posterior wall. In certain cases, the presence of septal kinking can invalidate the measurements.

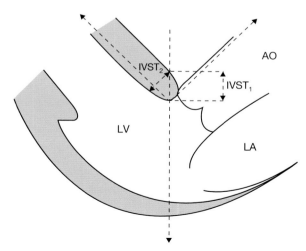

Figure 7.8   Septal kinking. Abnormal aortoseptal angle (< 90°) leading to an exaggerated measurement of the septal thickness ($IVST_1$). Normal septal thickness ($IVST_2$) reflecting the anatomical reality. AO, aorta; LA, left atrium; LV, left ventricle.

Pitfalls when calculating the left ventricular mass

LVH translates anatomically into an increase in the left ventricular mass (LVM). The LVM may be calculated using echocardiography:

- either with the M-mode measurements according to two recommended techniques (ASE and PENN; see Fig. 7.1 and Box 7.3)
- or by resorting to the 2D mode, which makes it possible to partially avoid the heterogeneous nature of the LV, but at a reproducibility that is too low to justify its complexity.

The most commonly used method for measuring the LVM is based on M-mode echocardiography. This method is relatively reliable for quantifying LVH, as it takes into account the wall thickness and the diameter of the ventricular chamber. It has been validated by anatomical correlations.

In reality, the size of the LV often varies, due to the variations in blood volume and load conditions, which renders the isolated measurement of the wall thicknesses insufficient for the quantification of hypertrophy.

Two formulae are commonly used to calculate the LVH in M-mode echocardiography: the ASE formula and the PENN/Devereux formula (see Box 7.3). These formulae are based on the common hypothesis of a LV that is geometrically a rotational ellipsoid truncated at one of its poles, and the major axis of which is double the length of the minor axis. In order to calculate the LVM, mathematical formulae based on the principle of cubes are used. It is nonetheless vital to match the chosen formula with the corresponding measurement convention being used.

In order to be reliable, the measurement of the M-mode parameters (thicknesses and diameter) used in calculating the mass must be rigorous and precise (see Fig. 7.2). However, echocardiographic measurement of the LVM may run into technical and methodological difficulties, and the examiner should be familiar with these in order to make an informed view of the final result (Box 7.4).

The pitfalls involved in calculating the LVM using M-mode echocardiography are described below.

Inappropriate use of the formulae for calculating the left ventricular mass

The formulae for calculating the LVM are valid only for elliptically shaped, morphologically homogeneous LVs. Moreover, it is vital to check which of the mathematical formulae is integrated in the calculation software of the ultrasound machine being used in order to apply the correct corresponding measurement technique (ASE or PENN convention). This makes it possible to avoid errors in the diagnosis of LVH.

Incorrect calculation of the myocardial mass

When the examination conditions are difficult, or in certain pathological situations, the elliptical model of the LV becomes inapplicable (see Box 7.4). The technical difficulties associated with obtaining a high-quality M-mode trace in

---

Box 7.4   Principal limitations in the calculation of the left ventricular mass using M-mode echocardiography

- Reduced patient echogenicity
- Subaortic septal rim
- Asymmetrical septal hypertrophy
- Paradoxical septal motion
- Regional wall motion abnormalities (ischaemic cardiopathy)
- Left ventricular dilatation (dilated cardiopathy)
- Deformation of the left ventricular chamber (aneurysm)
- Left bundle branch block of the His bundle

---

patients who have a low echogenicity constitute an overwhelming limitation on the precise measurement of the wall thicknesses.

Failure to respect the conditions of M-mode measurements (see Box 7.1)
In short, an echocardiographic methodology that is not rigorous gives rise to an unreliable result.

Errors due to 'cubing' of the ventricle
In practice, even a small error in measurement can have significant consequences, as the ventricular thicknesses and diameters are cubed. For example, for wall thicknesses of 12 mm and a diameter of 55 mm, a 1 mm overestimation of the thickness of the septum and the posterior wall lead to an error of 40 g in an LVM of 351 g.

Poor reproducibility of the left ventricular mass calculation
The coefficient of variation in the LVM calculation is around 20 g, or even 30 g. This generates an apparent spontaneous regression of the LVH over repeated examinations, linked to the phenomenon of regression to the mean.

Significant intra- and interobserver variability
Intra- and interobserver variability limits the reproducibility of the examination, and should cause examiners to be particularly careful in their interpretation of individual results. In the same patient, the comparison of two successive examinations or even readings made at two different moments during the same examination may lead to notable variation in the calculated LVM. For good reproducibility, in terms of intraobserver variability, differences of less than 1 mm in the measured wall thicknesses and of less than 2 mm in the measured chambers are vital. It is, therefore, sensible to make measurements over at least three cardiac cycles to obtain good reproducibility. The definitive values will then be the mean values.

Variability of threshold values used for the diagnosis of left ventricular hypertrophy

The parameters that significantly modify the LVM are the gender and the body habitus of the patient. As a matter of routine, the LVM is corrected according to the patient's body surface area, with an average threshold of 134 g/m² for men and 110 g/m² for women usually being applied. However, the threshold values proposed in the literature are somewhat variable: 110–134 g/m² for men and 100–125 g/m² for women.

Uncertainty over the choice of the threshold value has major consequences for the final diagnosis of LVH. By applying low thresholds, the overall prevalence of LVH is increased considerably. Therefore the choice of the thresholds for defining LVH has a significant influence on the estimated value of this prevalence. In contrast, an underestimation of LVH is observed in obese patients when relating the LVM to the body surface area. For this reason, indexing the LVM by patient size, preferably raised to the power of 2.7, has been proposed. In a normal subject, this index of the LVM should be lower than 50 g/m²·⁷ in men and 47 g/m²·⁷ in women. Generally, the thresholds determining the LVH are lower in women (Table 7.1).

Finally, in order to define the left ventricular geometry, the calculation of the LVM should be complemented by the corresponding measurement of the relative wall thickness (RWT). The RWT is expressed as:

$$\text{RWT} = \text{IVST} + \text{PWT/EDD} \ (n < 0.45)$$

This echocardiographic parameter, interpreted according to the corrected LVM, makes it possible to specify the concentric or eccentric character of the LVH, which is often a source of confusion (Table 7.2 and Fig. 7.9). In fact, even if the LVM is normal, an RWT of > 0.45 makes it possible to identify concentric

Table 7.1   Normal values of the left ventricular mass (LVM) indexed according to the body surface area and size of the patient

Indexed LVM	Men	Women
To body surface area (g/m²)	< 134	< 110
To size (g/m²·⁷)	< 50	< 47

Table 7.2   Three morphological types of abnormal left ventricular geometry

Abnormal geometry	Left ventricular mass (LVM)	Relative wall thickness (RWT)
Concentric remodelling	Normal	> 0.45
Eccentric LVH	Increased (↑)	< 0.45
Concentric LVH	Increased (↑↑)	> 0.45

LVH, left ventricular hypertrophy.

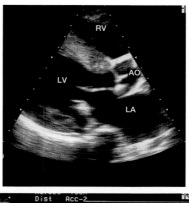

(a)

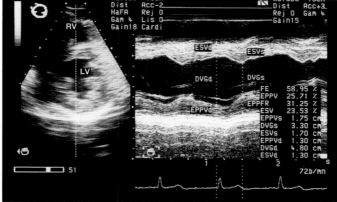

(b)

Figure 7.9   Concentric hypertrophy of the left ventriclular walls in 2D and M-mode echocardiography (diastolic wall thicknesses = 13 mm, relative wall thickness = 0.54). AO, aorta; LA, left atrium; LV, left ventricle; RV, right ventricle.

remodelling of the LV. The advantage of a morphological analysis of the geometry of the LV lies in its prognostic implications (stratification of the cardiovascular risk in hypertensive patients).

Finally, quantification of the LVM in 2D echocardiography on the basis of the myocardial contours has never been proved superior to M-mode measurement.

Preliminary data on the calculation of the LVM by means of three-dimensional echocardiography appear promising, particularly in cases of non-homogeneous hypertrophy.

DISTINCTION BETWEEN PHYSIOLOGICAL AND PATHOLOGICAL LEFT VENTRICULAR HYPERTROPHY

The regular practice of a sustained sporting activity is accompanied by morphological modifications of the LV, in particular an increase in the wall thicknesses. It is sometimes difficult to trace the exact border between 'physiological' hypertrophy linked to sport and pathological hypertrophy. The echocardiographic data that make it possible to distinguish between these two types of LVH are summarized in Table 7.3, where measurements of the heart of an athlete are compared with measurements found in hypertrophic cardiomyopathy (HCM). The application of DTI is very useful in this differential diagnosis.

Table 7.3   Differential diagnosis between physiological hypertrophy (athlete's heart) and pathological hypertrophy (hypertrophic cardiomyopathy (HCM))

Parameter	Athlete's heart	HCM
Wall thickness	< 13 mm (13–15 mm in 5% of cases)	≥ 13 mm
IVST/PWT	< 1.3	> 1.3
RWT	Variable	> 0.45
Left ventricular mass	Increased (↑)	Increased (↑↑)
EDD of the LV	≥ 55 mm (> 60 mm in 14% of cases)	< 50 mm
LV systolic function	Normal	Normal
Left ventricular diastolic function		
Mitral flow	E/A > 1 DT > 150 ms IVRT ≥ 90 ms	E/A < 1 or > 1 DT > 220 ms, IVRT > 90 ms
PV (colour M-mode)	> 45 cm/s	< 45 cm/s
Ea (annular DTI)	> 8 cm/s	< 8 cm/s
Filling pressure	Normal	Normal or increased
Myocardial DTI		
Myocardial velocities	Normal	Reduced
Transparietal gradient	Normal	Increased
Intra-LV dynamic obstruction	Absent	Often present
Mitral regurgitation	Absent or small	Moderate
Pulmonary arterial pressures	Normal	Normal or increased
Evolution	Regression of the hypertrophy with loss of fitness	Persistence of hypertrophy

DT, deceleration time; DTI, Doppler tissue imaging; Ea, velocity of the E wave in DTI applied to the mitral annulus; E/A, ratio of the E and A waves of the mitral flow; IVRT, isovolumic relaxation time; IVST/PWT, ratio of the septal diastolic thicknesses to the posterior wall thickness; LV, left ventricle; PV, propagation velocity of the mitral flow in colour M-mode; RWT, relative wall thickness; EDD, end-diastolic diameter of the LV.

PITFALLS WHEN DIAGNOSING PRIMARY HYPERTROPHIC CARDIOMYOPATHY

Hypertrophic cardiomyopathy (HCM) is the most frequently occurring of the monogenic hereditary cardiopathies. Typically it is characterized by a disproportionate hypertrophy of the LV with or without dynamic outflow back obstruction. Doppler echocardiography is considered to be the diagnostic method of choice for HCM, but the results are is sometimes difficult to interpret, and all the more so if the condition is highly heterogeneous.

The diagnostic difficulties and potential pitfalls when using the Doppler technique relate to:

- the early diagnosis of HCM
- the location and degree of the wall hypertrophy
- the detection of a dynamic intraventricular obstruction
- the distinction between the HCM and the subaortic septal rim (Table 7.4)
- HCM associated with arterial hypertension
- the coexistence of aortic stenosis with HCM
- the distinction between HCM and LVH in a high-level sportsperson (see Table 7.3)
- HCM in the elderly
- the differential diagnosis between Fabry's disease, a systemic condition and a cardiac tumour
- hypertrophic pseudocardiomyopathy due to a congenital malformation.

Table 7.4 Differential diagnosis between the subaortic septal rim and hypertrophic obstructive cardiomyopathy (HOCM)

Parameter	Septal rim	HOCM
Clinical context	Older, often hypertensive subject	Younger subject, familial primary HOCM
Septal hypertrophy	Located on the basal septum	More diffuse, surrounding the middle segment of the septum
Diastolic septal thickness	13–20 mm	Often > 20 mm
Septal echostructure	Normal	Hyperechoic, dense appearance
Septal motion	Normal	Hypokinetic
Left ventricle	Normal size	Small, deformed
Dynamic obstruction	Rare (around 18% of cases)	Frequent (> 50% of cases)
Diastolic function	Conserved	Altered

Early diagnosis of hypertrophic cardiomyopathy

The appearance of ventricular hypertrophy in carriers of a familial form of HCM is often delayed. In fact, around 30% of carriers of the genetic mutation present no cardiac hypertrophy. Standard echocardiography does not therefore make it possible to identify those patients with the mutation but without hypertrophy. In contrast, DTI allows early detection of the myocardial anomalies in patients affected by HCM, even before the hypertrophy arises. It shows, above all, a significant reduction in the systolic and diastolic myocardial velocities in carriers of the genetic mutation.

Location and degree of wall hypertrophy

In its usual form, LVH is generally asymmetrical, predominating in 90% of all cases over the subaortic part of the interventricular septum (Fig. 7.10). The measurement of the thickness of the walls, in particular the septal wall, requires

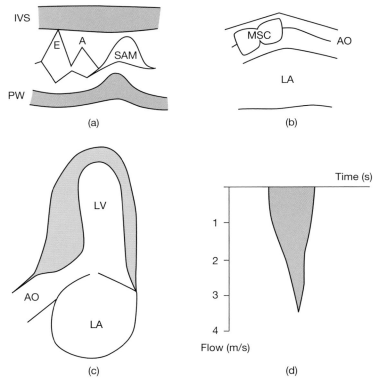

Figure 7.10 Echo Doppler anomalies of hypertrophic obstructive cardiomyopathy. (a) Abnormal systolic anterior motion (SAM) of the mitral valve in M-mode. (b) Partial midsystolic closure (MSC) of the aortic valve in M-mode. (c) Subaortic septal hypertrophy in 2D apical cross-section. (d) Intra-left ventricular dynamic obstruction flow in continuous Doppler. AO, aorta; IVS, interventricular septum; LA, left atrium; LV, left ventricle; PW, posterior wall.

considerable rigour (see Table 7.1). The arbitrary nature of the diagnostic thresh-old values determines the sensitivity of echocardiography. The septal thickness required for echocardiographic diagnosis of the sporadic forms of HCM is ≥ 15 mm during diastole (Fig. 7.11). In genetic studies, the most commonly accepted threshold value is 13 mm, in order to increase the sensitivity of detect-ing familial forms of HCM (at the expense of specificity). A septum/posterior wall thickness ratio of > 1.5 is more specific, but less sensitive than the figure of 1.3, and is considered an alternative diagnostic value.

A hypertrophied septum is typically hypokinetic or akinetic, and is highly echogenic (ground-glass appearance) in cases of HCM.

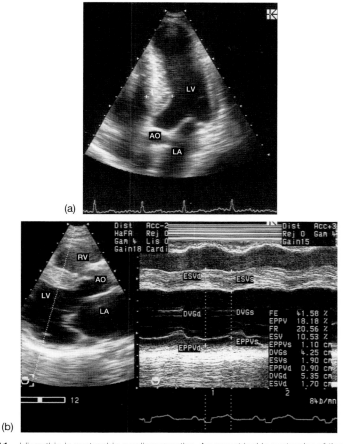

Figure 7.11   Idiopathic hypertrophic cardiomyopathy. Asymmetrical hypertrophy of the left ventricle (LV) predominating over the subaortic part of the hypokinetic and highly echogenic interventricular septum (diastolic septal thickness 17 mm). AO, aorta; LA, left atrium; RV, right ventricle.

In addition to the classical forms of HCM with asymmetric septal hypertrophy, the hypertrophy may be:

- midventricular
- apical
- anterolateral
- extending into the right ventricle.

This atypical distribution of the hypertrophy should be identified using the 2D mode, and all possible echocardiographic projections in order to avoid diagnostic errors. The operator should search systematically for a hypertrophy associated with the right ventricle. Finally, it should be noted that the causes of asymmetrical septal hypertrophy may be numerous (Table 7.5). These causes should, therefore, be discussed during the interpretation of the echocardiographic findings according to the clinical context.

Detection of left ventricular outflow obstruction

HCM is a potential cause of outflow obstruction during left ventricular ejection. This obstruction, generally located in the subaortic area (in the left ventricular outflow chamber, between the septum and the mitral valve), can be seen in Doppler echocardiography through:

- the systolic anterior motion (SAM) of the mitral valvular and subvalvular apparatus towards the interventricular septum, visualized using M-mode and 2D (see Fig. 7.11);
- the partial midsystolic closure (MSC) of the aortic valve, recorded in M-mode

Table 7.5   Possible causes of asymmetrical septal hypertrophy (ASH)

Age group	Causes
Newborn	Physiological
Child	Any obstruction to the right or left ventricular ejection (congenital aortic stenosis, aortic coarctation)
	Pulmonary arterial hypertension
	Tumour of the heart
Adult	Sporting activity (athlete's/physiological hypertrophy)
	Aortic stenosis
	Arterial hypertension
	Infarct of the lower myocardium (compensatory reactionary ASH)
	Older age (subaortic septal rim)
	Persistent congenital malformation
	Systemic illness (cardiac amyloid)
	Infiltrative tumour of the heart

- the left ventricular outflow pressure gradient, evaluated using continuous Doppler.

The echocardiographic pitfalls when diagnosing outflow obstruction due to HCM are summarized in Box 7.5. These are principally technical limitations in the complete recording of the high outflow velocity, which makes it possible to measure the intra-left ventricular pressure gradient, reflecting the severity of the ventricular outflow obstruction (Fig. 7.12). In practice, the maximum gradient is retained, as the mean gradient has less meaning given the asymmetrical evolution of the flow. The obstruction is considered severe if the pressure gradient is > 50 mmHg.

The left ventricular outflow obstruction may be recorded using continuous Doppler coupled with 2D imaging once the level of the obstruction has been detected (aliasing) using 2D colour Doppler (see Fig. 7.12). However, this obstruction is often very localized and requires a stand-alone 'blind' search of the maximum velocities using the Pedoff-type probe (without coupled imaging), which can be manipulated with ease. The spectrum recorded using continuous Doppler must be clear and well defined in order to be valid.

Finally, the left ventricular outflow obstruction identified using continuous Doppler should be distinguished from the systolic flow of mitral regurgitation, particularly as the latter is associated with HOCM in over 50% of cases (Table 7.6).

Box 7.5   Echocardiographic pitfalls in diagnosing dynamic obstruction in hypertrophic cardiomyopathy (HCM)

- Technical limitations:
  - poor quality of the M-mode trace, making it impossible to visualize the SAM and/or the MSC
  - non-optimal alignment of the Doppler beam with the obstructive flow, leading to an underestimation of the gradient
- Limited specificity of the SAM and MSC:
  - false SAM (hyperkinetic syndromes, acute hypovolaemia, tamponade, mitral prolapse, subvalvular aortic stenosis, in postmitral valvuloplasty, after valve replacement for aortic stenosis, mitral slit, malpositioning of the chordae or papillary muscles
  - other causes of MSC (low output, mitral prolapse, aortic dissection, subvalvular aortic stenosis, high septal interventricular communication)
- Possible confusion between the obstruction flow and the mitral regurgitation flow
- Absence of dynamic obstruction:
  - in basal state (in 50–70% of HCM)
  - in apical forms of HCM
- Failure to carry out a provocative test enabling the possible induction of the dynamic obstruction
- Systolodiastolic dynamic obstruction (midventricular HCM)

MSC, midsystolic closure; SAM, systolic anterior motion.

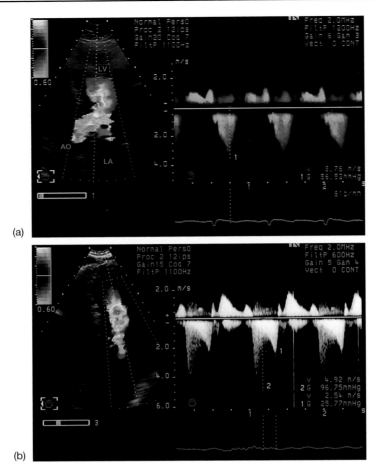

Figure 7.12 Hypertrophic obstructive cardiomyopathy. Examples of subaortic dynamic obstruction identified using 2D colour and continuous Doppler. Maximum left intraventricular systolic pressure gradient: (a) 56 mmHg; (b) 26 mmHg. (b) Superimposition of the associated obstructive and mitral regurgitation flows. AO, aorta; LA, left atrium; LV, left ventricle.

The mitral regurgitation may have a similar shape and be superimposed on the obstructive flow (Fig. 7.13). However, the regurgitated flow is larger, of a higher velocity and has an earlier peak. Unlike the obstructive flow, it includes periods of isovolumic contraction and relaxation of the LV. This element is important in the differential diagnosis between the two flows. Colour Doppler is helpful in discerning between these two systolic velocity profiles.

With regard to the SAM, it is not pathognomonic of HCM. In fact, it may be found in other circumstances without wall hypertrophy (see Box 7.5). This false SAM is usually early systolic, whereas the SAM of HCM is midsystolic at most. Likewise, MSC is also found in other conditions, where it occurs during early or end-systole (see Box 7.4).

Table 7.6 Differential diagnosis between the obstructive flow of hypertrophic cardiomyopathy and mitral regurgitation in continuous and colour Doppler

Characteristic	Obstructive flow	Mitral regurgitation
Continuous Doppler		
Morphology	Dagger shaped	Symmetrical
Crest	Pointed and delayed	Rounded
Peak	End-systolic	Mid-systolic
Maximum velocity	3–6 m/s	> 4 m/s
Beginning	Later (during aortic opening)	In early systole (from mitral closing)
End	Aortic closing	Mitral opening
2D colour Doppler		
Appearance of flow	Aliased intra-LV ejection flow	Intra-LA mitral regurgitation flow, more or less aliased

LA, left atrium; LV, left ventricle.

The left intraventricular dynamic obstruction may be permanent, labile (the gradient varying over time) or latent. It may be provoked by the following tests:

- Valsalva manoeuvre
- pharmacodynamic tests (glyceryl trinitrate, Isuprel, amyl nitrite)
- exercise echocardiography.

These provocative tests allow the detection of a left ventricular outflow obstruction that is absent or low in the basal state (i.e. while resting).

Certain particularities of dynamic obstructions are due to the atypical forms of HCM. In the presence of a midventricular hypertrophy, the LV is separated into two chambers during systole, one basal and the other apical. In the apical chamber the higher pressures may lead in the long term to a necrosis of the apex. The necrotic apical region becomes akinetic or dyskinetic, and the pressure gradient becomes uncharacteristic. In this case, Doppler echocardiography can be used to show the intraventricular gradient, both systolic and diastolic. The systolic obstruction located at the level of the hypertrophied papillary muscles (Fig. 7.14) appears as a result of the muscular occlusion, and not on contact between the mitral valve and the septum. The diastolic part of the obstruction seems to be due to the delay in relaxation of the midventricular zone, even as the apex, where the pressures are still high, continues to empty towards the base of the LV.

The apical form of the HCM is typical of a diagnostic pitfall: only using 2D echocardiography it is possible to detect the complete hypertrophy of the apex of the LV, which is obliterated during systole. This apical form of HCM is not usually accompanied by any left intraventricular gradient, whether in the basal state or after pharmacological provocation. The SAM is also absent.

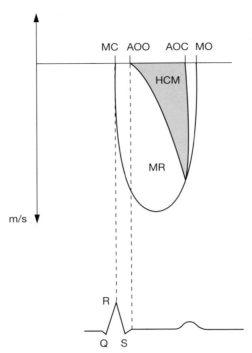

Figure 7.13 Dagger-shaped morphology of the obstructed flow due to hypertrophic cardiomyopathy (HCM) and the rounded appearance of mitral regurgitation (MR) flow. Superimposition of the two flows picked up in continuous Doppler from the apex with a simultaneous electrocardiogram. The isovolumic contraction time is respected in the case of HCM. AOC, aortic closing; AOO, aortic opening; MC, mitral closing; MO, mitral opening.

Box 7.6 Possible causes of a left ventricular outflow obstruction other than hypertrophic cardiomyopathy

- Normal subjects in hypovolaemia
- Concentric left ventricular hypertrophy, with a small ventricular chamber
- Obstructive subaortic septal rim
- Systemic illness: cardiac amyloidosis
- During cardiac tamponade (inspiratory crushing of the left ventricle)
- Following cardiac valve surgery (valve replacement due to aortic stenosis, mitral plasty)
- Certain congenital cardiopathies (transposition of the large vessels, subvalvular aortic stenosis, etc.)
- During stress echocardiography

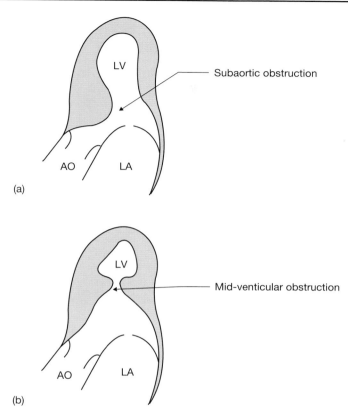

Figure 7.14   Two types of left intraventricular dynamic obstruction. (a) Subaortic obstruction located in the left ventricular outflow chamber (due to subaortic septal hypertrophy). (b) Mid-ventricular obstruction located at the level of the hypertrophic papillary muscles. AO, aorta; LA, left atrium; LV, left ventricle.

LVH may predominate at the level of the posterior wall, leaving the septal wall free (inverted asymmetrical hypertrophy). In this case, the left ventricular outflow chamber is stenotic and SAM is visible in the majority of cases. A dynamic obstruction is visible in continuous Doppler in approximately 60% of cases.

Finally, other possible causes of left ventricular outflow obstruction should be eliminated (Box 7.6). In these situations, the obstruction is generally midventricular, without a SAM.

It should also be noted that HOCM is frequently accompanied by a small positive flow (in the opposite direction to the obstructive flow) of low velocity, arising during the period of isovolumic relaxation of the LV. This flow appears to correspond to asynchronous relaxation of the apical and basal parts of the septum, creating a local pressure gradient that leads to a movement of blood towards the apex of the LV.

Special cases

Hypertrophic cardiomyopathy associated with arterial hypertension

Several elements make it difficult to distinguish between HOCM associated with an arterial hypertension and LVH secondary to an arterial hypertension. This problem arises predominantly in older hypertensive subjects. In fact, a genuine intraventricular obstruction may exist in certain marked forms: hypertensive hypertrophic cardiomyopathies. The causes of a possible dynamic obstruction in the older hypertensive patient in particular are:

- a concentric hypertrophy of the LV with a small ventricular chamber
- an asymmetrical hypertrophy of the LV in the form of an obstructive sub-aortic septal rim (see Table 7.4).

In practice, identifying this group of patients is important, as a vasodilator and/or diuretic treatment could possibly aggravate their symptoms.

Hypertrophic cardiomyopathy in older subjects

Certain echocardiographic characteristics are associated with the forms of HCM seen in elderly patients. The findings that make it possible to distinguish HCM in the elderly from that seen in younger patients are:

- the smaller size of the wall hypertrophy
- the high incidence of a dynamic obstruction (60–80% of cases)
- a frequent distortion of the LV (reversal of the septal curvature, crescent shaped)
- coexistence of a calcified mitral ring.

In fact, the association of a hypertrophy of the basal septum and a calcified mitral ring in an older patient lead to a predisposition towards dynamic obstruction due to stenosis of the left ventricular outflow chamber.

Hypertrophic cardiomyopathy and Fabry's disease

Fabry's disease is a chromosomal disorder leading to an accumulation of sphingolipids in various tissues, such as the myocardium. It may be isolated (cardiac variant of the disease) or integrated into a systemic form. Cardiac hypertrophy due to Fabry's disease may mimic HCM, and should therefore be systematically searched for in every patient with an unexplained ventricular cardiomyopathy.

However, this hypertrophy is generally homogeneous and symmetrical. The echo structure of the myocardium is usually unchanged. The advantage of early diagnosis of Fabry's disease is that it becomes possible to implement specific treatment with substitute enzyme therapy.

Hypertrophic cardiomyopathy and systemic diseases

Certain systemic diseases, such as amyloidosis or haemochromatosis, may lead to hypertrophy of the heart as a result of myocardial infiltration (Fig. 7.15).

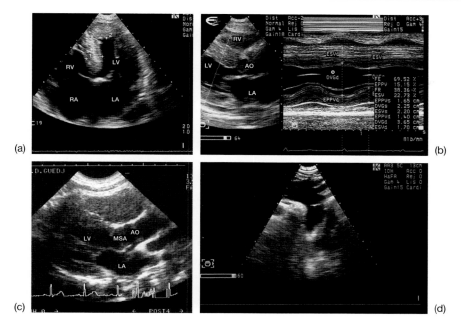

Figure 7.15   Particular cases of left ventricular hypertrophy (LVH). (a, b) Cardiac amyloid: hypertrophic and hyperechoic septoapical wall (note the tiny pericardial effusion). (c, d) Congenital malformations leading to LVH: (c) subaortic diaphragm; (d) aortic coarctation. AO, aorta; LA, left atrium; LV, left ventricle; MSA, mitral surface area; RA, right atrium; RV, right ventricle.

Echocardiography makes it possible to detect a wall hypertrophy of variable size, uni- or biventricular, which may be responsible for a dynamic obstruction in certain isolated cases. This form of myocardial involvement should be distinguished from HOCM.

Echocardiographic anomalies of systemic diseases affecting the heart are non-specific in isolation, but their association is often highly suggestive of a myocardial infiltration, such as amyloid (hyperechoic and heterogeneous, ground-glass appearance of the hypertrophic myocardium).

Hypertrophic cardiomyopathy and cardiac tumours
An asymmetrical septal hypertrophy may be due to a heart tumour, in particular a septally located rhabdomyoma. The diagnosis of this tumour is made in the context of Bourneville's tuberous sclerosis and the hyperechoic appearance of the tumour.

Hypertrophic pseudocardiomyopathy
The presence of a fixed subaortic stenosis (e.g. in the form of a membrane) may lead to an asymmetrical septal hypertrophy, known as 'reactional', that simulates HCM (hypertrophic pseudocardiomyopathy).

However, a careful 2D echocardiographic examination of the left ventricular outflow chamber will make it possible to identify the fixed subaortic obstruction. Colour Doppler will confirm an acceleration of the ejection flow of the LV on contact with this obstruction.

PITFALLS WHEN DIAGNOSING MYOCARDIAL ISCHAEMIA

Doppler echocardiography is playing an increasing role in the assessment of patients presenting with ischaemic cardiomyopathy. The echocardiographic analysis of the contractility of a ventricular wall requires the dual evaluation of:

- the amplitude of the excursion of the endocardium during systole
- the systolic thickening of the wall.

These two parameters are best measured using the M-mode technique, with the ultrasound beam perpendicular to the walls. Unfortunately, only the septal and basal posterior walls of the LV are analysed using this technique. A complete regional study of the ventricular walls requires the use of 2D echocardiography. However, 2D analysis of the regional motion of the LV has its own technical problems and diagnostic limitations (Box 7.7). Firstly, the analysis is purely visual, subjective and qualitative. Secondly, it requires visualization of different ventricular segments through the use of multiple, high-quality, 2D cross-sections. In practice, the segmental contractility of the LV is examined in a comparative manner, segment by segment, in order to identify a contractile asynergy that can be manifested in three forms (Fig. 7.16):

- hypokinesia – insufficient contraction
- akinesia – absence of contraction
- dyskinesia – paradoxical contractions.

The precise definition of these abnormal contractions is summarized in Table 7.7. However, the diagnosis of abnormal ventricular contractions (Fig. 7.17) using conventional echocardiography may be imprecise, difficult or impossible in

---

Box 7.7   Echocardiographic pitfalls relating to the analysis of the segmental motion of the left ventricle

- Poor quality of the M-mode and/or 2D image (patient hypoechogenicity, incorrect adjustment of the ultrasound machine, lack of harmonic technology, etc.)

- Insufficient experience of the examiner

- Failure to use multiple echocardiographic projections (incomplete analysis of all the ventricular segments)

- Imprecise or incorrect interpretation of the state of the wall motion

- Subjectivity in the evaluation of the wall contractility

- Lack of reliable quantitative criteria for abnormal contractions

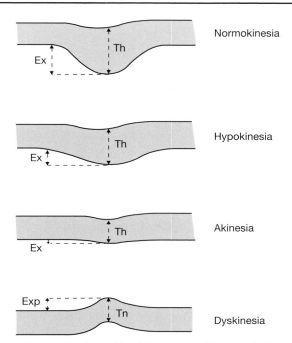

Figure 7.16   Normal wall motion (normokinesia) and contractile anomalies (hypokinesia, akinesia, dyskinesia). Ex, endocardial excursion; Exp, paradoxical expansion; Th, systolic thickening; Tn, systolic thinning.

Table 7.7   Definition of normal segmental motion (normokinesia) and contractile anomalies (hypokinesia, akinesia, dyskinesia)

Motion type	Defining characteristics
Normokinesia	Endocardial excursion > 5 mm Systolic thickening ≥ 50%
Hypokinesia	Endocardial excursion 2–5 mm Systolic thickening < 50%
Akinesia	Endocardial excursion 0–2 mm Absence of systolic thickening
Dyskinesia	Paradoxical expansion in systole Absence of thickening, or even systolic thinning

certain situations. This method suffers principally from the difficulties of precisely delineating the ventricular endocardium.

The analysis of the ventricular contractility of an ischaemic cardiomyopathy may be improved by the application of complementary echocardiographic techniques such as:

- harmonic imaging
- stress echocardiography
- colour kinesis
- myocardial DTI (Fig. 7.18)
- myocardial contrast echocardiography.

In future, three-dimensional echocardiography will also have a role to play in this field, particularly with matrix probes making it possible to measure the cardiac volumes over the course of a single cardiac cycle.

Echocardiographic pitfalls when diagnosing myocardial infarction

The echocardiographic diagnosis of myocardial infarction (MI) is based on the demonstration of a segmental myocardial dysfunction. It is important to know the limits of the echocardiographic technique, as well as the pitfalls relating to the diagnosis (Box 7.8). In fact, the segmental dysfunction, associating an impaired excursion of the endocardium (reduced, suppressed, or even paradoxical) with a reduced thickening of the wall, arises for a transmural extension of the infarction of > 20%. It is present very early in > 90% of patients in the acute phase of transmural infarction. The asynergic zone of the infarcted territory usually contrasts with the compensatory hyperkinesia of the non-ischaemic segments opposite the necrosis.

In contrast, the segments adjacent to the infarcted zone are frequently hypokinetic due to the intervention of a mechanical, rather than an ischaemic, disorder, due to their proximity to the infarcted zone (stretching phenomenon).

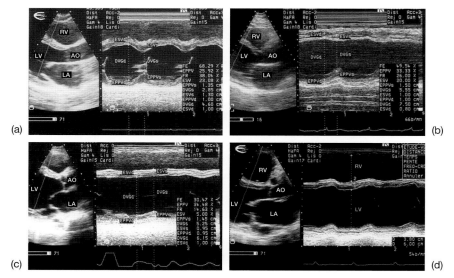

Figure 7.17 Left ventricular wall motion evaluated using M-mode on the basis of the parasternal, long-axis cross-section: (a) normokinesia; (b) septal hypokinesia; (c) septal akinesia; (d) septal dyskinesia. AO, aorta; LA, left atrium; V, left ventricle; RV, right ventricle.

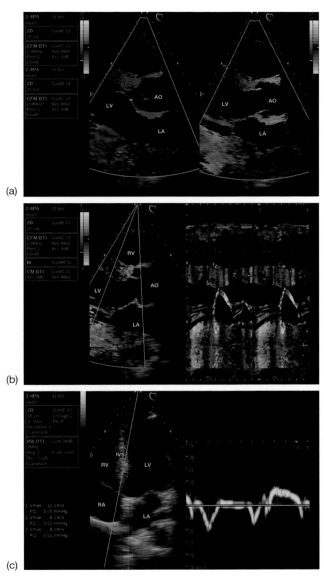

Figure 7.18   Normal Doppler tissue imaging (Imagic system, Kontron-Esaote) in 2D mode. (a) Visual analysis of the left ventricular wall motion, the intramyocardial velocities of which are colour coded. Apical cross-section of the four chambers: images during diastole (left) and systole (right). (b) In M-mode and the parasternal long-axis cross-section. M-mode analysis of the temporal evaluation of the myocardial velocities and their spatial distribution over the length of the cardiac cycle. (c) In spectral mode. Recording of pulsed Doppler signal in the septal wall of the left ventricle (LV). Normal triphasic appearance of the spectrum: two negative waves during diastole (11 and 8 cm/s) followed by a positive wave during systole (8 cm/s). AO, aorta; LA, left atrium; RA, right atrium; RV, right ventricle; IVS, interventricular septum.

So-called 'distant' zones may also be asynergic. This is generally due to an ischaemia linked to subendocardial microinfarctions.

However, a ventricular asynergy visualized using echocardiography may not correspond to an infarction. The causes of false-positive diagnoses (non-specific motion anomalies) are summarized in Box 7.9. In fact, no akinetic or hypo-kinetic wall is necessarily necrotic (stunning or hibernation phenomenon, primitive disorder, focal myocarditis, etc.). Moreover, a paradoxical septal motion is possible apart from ischaemia. In cases of infarction without ST segment elevation on the ECG, the contractile anomalies are inconsistent and a normal ECG

Box 7.8   Echocardiographic pitfalls when diagnosing myocardial infarction

- Pitfalls due to the analysis of the segmental motion of the left ventricle (see Box 7.7)
- Diagnoses by default or through excess of the infarction (see Box 7.9)
- Imprecise evaluation of the location and extent of the infarction
- Difficulties in the objective evaluation of the severity of the necrosis
- Non-diagnosis of post-infarction left ventricular remodelling
- Possible unfamiliarity with certain complications of infarction (septal rupture, papillary muscle rupture, mural thrombus, etc.)
- Sometimes, difficulty in distinguishing between:
  - a mitral regurgitation secondary to the remodelling and an ischaemic mitral regurgitation
  - a left ventricular aneurysm and a false aneurysm
- Possible reversibility of the asynergies following myocardial revascularization

---

Box 7.9   Causes of false-negative and false-positive diagnoses of myocardial infarction

False-negative diagnoses
- Non-transmural infarction
- Small size of infarction, particularly in a posterior location
- Infarction affecting the right ventricular walls, which are difficult to analyse

False-positive diagnoses
- Technical cause (tangential projection)
- Ischaemic cause without infarction (threat syndrome, Prinzmetal's angina)
- Where myocardial viability is present (stunning or hibernation effect)
- Cases of paradoxical septal motion of non-ischaemic origin (right ventricular overload, left beam branch block, postoperative (coronary bridging, valve replacement, etc.))
- Incipient non-ischaemic myocardial attack

does not rule out the diagnosis of MI. Finally, chronic myocardial ischaemia, like the infarction, may also be a source of segmental contraction anomalies.

Location and extent of the infarction

The location of the infarction should be found using echocardiography by means of a careful analysis of all the ventricular segments, using, for example, the ASE's 17-segment model (Fig. 7.19). This analysis, carried out in multiple 2D projections, makes it possible to obtain diagnostic information about the patient's coronary disorder. This information, however, should be interpreted with some caution. In fact, there is an ambiguity of coronary distribution for the apical section of the inferior wall and the lateral wall, which may lead to errors in determining the location of the coronary lesion. Where the infarction is in its acute phase, the initial extent of ventriculat dysfunction is well correlated with the zone at risk, i.e. the zone threatened with necrosis in the absence of reperfusion. In contrast, after effective reperfusion, the asynergic zone identified on echocardiography overestimates the true size of the infarction, as a part of this zone corresponds to stunned myocardium. A quantitative analysis of the regional left ventricular function in 2D echocardiography, based on the calculation of the wall motion score, is increasingly used, thanks to progress in information technology. This enables an evaluation of the severity of the myocardial ischaemia. However, the scoring method routinely used is based on a visual evaluation of the regional contractility. It is best carried out by re-reading the 2D echocardiographic projections. This method is reliable and reproducible in experienced users, although it suffers, nonetheless, as a result of its subjectivity.

Postinfarction left ventricular remodelling

The remodelling reflects the adaptation of the LV to the loss of part of its contractile potential. An expansion of the necrotic zone is associated with a dilatation of the healthy zone, followed by a compensatory wall hypertrophy. This ventricular remodelling, exclusively involving transmural MIs, must be identified early using echocardiography, as it is one of the major determining factors in prognosis.

Complications of the infarction

Echocardiography makes it possible to seek out certain complications of the infarction. This search must be systematic and, more particularly, concentrated on the mechanical complications (free wall or septal rupture, rupture of a papillary muscle), ischaemic mitral regurgitation and mural thrombi.

However, the distinction between a mitral regurgitation secondary to ventricular remodelling and a more serious ischaemic mitral regurgitation is sometimes difficult (Table 7.8). Exercise echocardiography makes it possible to confirm the dynamic nature of ischaemic mitral insufficiencies (see page 92). Likewise, it is vital to differentiate between left ventricular aneurysm complicating the infarction and a false aneurysm secondary to myocardial rupture in the isolated pericardium. The ventricular aneurysm produces a 2D image of a dyskinetic or akinetic pocket, deforming the contour of the LV during diastole (Fig. 7.20). The false aneurysm appears in echocardiography in the form of a pocket, sometimes expansive during systole, which may contain a thrombus and which communicates with the ventricular chamber through a narrow neck. Apical thrombi complicating anterior transmural infarctions should be differentiated from apical trabeculations or false tendons (Fig. 7.21). The use of harmonic imaging and contrast agents allows an improvement in their detection.

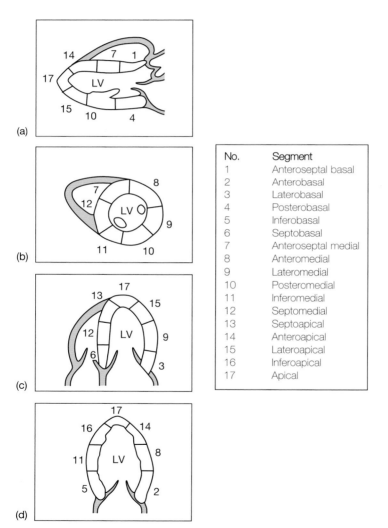

No.	Segment
1	Anteroseptal basal
2	Anterobasal
3	Laterobasal
4	Posterobasal
5	Inferobasal
6	Septobasal
7	Anteroseptal medial
8	Anteromedial
9	Lateromedial
10	Posteromedial
11	Inferomedial
12	Septomedial
13	Septoapical
14	Anteroapical
15	Lateroapical
16	Inferoapical
17	Apical

Figure 7.19 Segmentation of the left ventricular walls according to different echocardiographic cross-sections: (a) parasternal long-axis; (b) transverse parasternal; (c) apical four chamber; (d) apical two chamber. LV, left ventricle.

Table 7.8   Distinction between mitral regurgitation (MR) secondary to remodelling of the left ventricle (LV) and ischaemic MR due to papillary muscle dysfunction

Characteristic	Remodelling MR	Ischaemic MR
Causes	Geometric modifications of the LV chamber	Ventricular remodelling overall and regional LV dysfunction
		Dilatation of the mitral annulus
Mechanisms	Lateral and posterior displacement of the papillary muscles	Valve restriction
		Incomplete closing of the mitral valve
Frequency	High	More rare
Degree	Low to moderate	Moderate to major
Location	Central	More or less eccentric

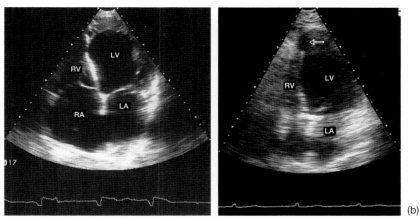

(a) (b)

Figure 7.20   Aneurysms of the left ventricle (LV) seen in the apical cross-section of the four chambers: (a) large aneurismal apical zone carpeted with a thrombus; (b) small aneurysm of the apex of the LV. LA, left atrium; RA, right atrium; RV, right ventricle.

PITFALLS WHEN DIAGNOSING PERICARDIAL LESIONS

The possibe pitfalls when diagnosing pericardial lesions are, above all:

- the detection and quantification of the pericardial effusion
- the identification of the cardiac tamponade
- the diagnosis of a constrictive chronic pericarditis.

Pitfalls in diagnosing effusive pericarditis
Echocardiography has become the diagnostic technique of choice for effusive pericarditis. The diagnosis of pericardial effusion is based on the presence of

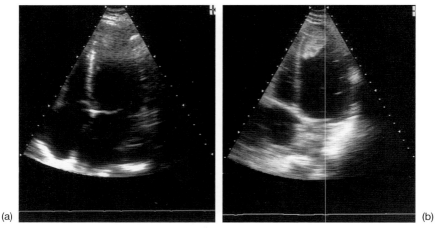

(a)   (b)

Figure 7.21 Post-infarction apical thrombi: (a) small thrombus, recent, low echogenicity; (b) voluminous thrombus located in the septoapical wall of the left ventricle.

an echo-free zone (clear space) between the epicardium and the pericardium. A significant pericardial effusion is characterized in M-mode echocardiography (parasternal, long-axis projection) by a systolodiastolic epicardial–pericardial separation, with a straightness of the pericardium, which tends to lose its mobility (Figs 7.22 and 7.23). In the 2D mode, all the echocardiographic projections are useful when looking for a pericardial effusion. The pitfalls of Doppler

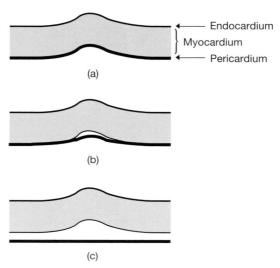

Figure 7.22 Three aspects of the epicardial–pericardial complex identifiable in M-mode echocardiography. (a) Normal aspect (absence of clear space). (b) Normal variant (purely systolic clear space, mobile pericardium). (c) Significant effusion (systolodiastolic separation, straight pericardium).

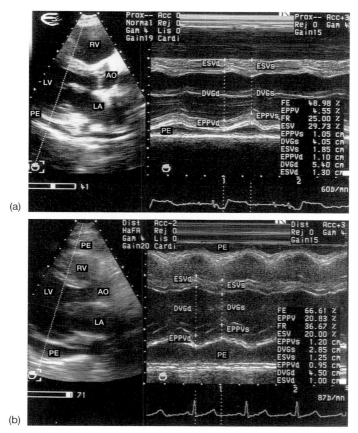

Figure 7.23 Examples of pericardial effusion (PE): (a) posterior, small; (b) average, non-compressive circumferential. AO, aorta; LA, left atrium; LV, left ventricle; RV, right ventricle.

echocardiography regarding the detection and quantification of the pericardial effusion are summarized in Box 7.10.

Diagnostic pitfalls

In order to confirm the presence of pericardial effusion by echocardiography, it is necessary to eliminate the causes of overdiagnosis and underdiagnosis. In fact, a purely systolic epicardial–pericardial separation, with the pericardium retaining its mobility, should be considered physiological (a variant of the norm) (see Fig. 7.22).

Causes of overdiagnosis of pericardial effusion

The main causes of overdiagnosis of pericardial effusion concern principally pericardial fat simulating effusive pericarditis, and pleural effusion that is possibly confused with pericardial effusion. In fact, an anterior isolated peri-cardial separation in the right ventricle is generally due to retrosternal peri-

---

> **Box 7.10   Echocardiographic pitfalls relating to the detection and quantification of pericardial effusion**
>
> - Errors of overdiagnosis:
>   - purely systolic pericardial separation with a mobile pericardium
>   - retrosternal pericardial fat
>   - pleural effusion
>   - ascites
>   - dilated coronary sinus
>   - mediastinal and pericardial tumours
>   - intrapericardial haematoma
>   - pericardial cysts
> - Errors of underdiagnosis:
>   - isolated or encapsulated pericardial effusion
>   - tiny non-detectable effusions in cases of 'dry' pericarditis
> - Association of the pericardial effusion with the pleural effusion
> - Semi-quantification of the abundance of the effusion
> - Echocardiographic identification of the cardiac tamponade
> - Possible extension of the abundant pericardial effusion towards the oblique pericardial sinus

cardial fat. It is fairly weak and particularly common in women, the obese and diabetics. The pericardial fat is rarely responsible for a posterior separation. In the case of any doubt, the nature of the dissection can be specified by means of a computed tomography (CT) scan or magnetic resonance imaging (MRI).

Pericardial effusion has an echocardiographic appearance that is often difficult to differentiate from a left pleural effusion. However, the latter is found not only behind the LV, but also behind the left atrium, which is not the case for pericardial effusion (Fig. 7.24).

In 2D, the position of the descending thoracic aorta in relation to the effusion is the determining factor: a pericardial effusion produces a preaortic clear space, while the left pleural effusion is retroaortic in the parasternal long-axis view (Fig. 7.25). When they are associated, the pericardial line separates the pleural effusion from the pericardial effusion.

Right pleural effusion is better visualized in the subcostal cross-section, where it is located behind the junction of the lower vena cava in the right atrium.

Echocardiographic confusion between ascites and pericardial effusion is rare. In fact, ascites is identifiable by means of the subcostal route in the presence of the falciform ligament of the liver at the centre of the effusion.

2D echocardiography can also be used to distinguish between pericardial effusion and a pathologically dilated coronary sinus, situated at the atrioventricular junction.

The differential diagnosis between pericardial effusion and mediastinal or pericardial tumours is best carried out using transoesophageal echocardiography

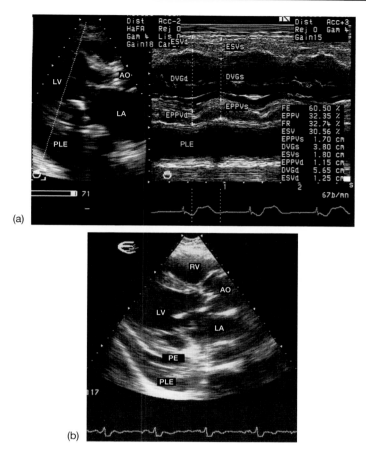

Figure 7.24   (a) Retroaortic left pleural effusion (PLE). (b) Small pericardial effusion (PE) separated from the pleural effusion by the pericardial line. AO, aorta; LA, left atrium; LV, left ventricle; RV, right ventricle.

(TEE). In the case of any doubt, thoracic scanning or MRI will allow a diagnosis to be made in the majority of cases.

Intrapericardial haematoma is found predominantly after surgery. It is often in a right retroatrial location. The pericardial cyst creates a clear space, usually adjoining the right atrium.

Causes of underdiagnosis of pericardial effusion

The causes of underdiagnosis of pericardial effusion are principally isolated or enclosed effusions in unusual locations (lateral or apical). These forms of the effusion are missed in M-mode echocardiography, but are identifiable in 2D echocardiography by using multiple projections. TEE is helpful in the diagnosis of these loculated effusions, which are located particularly at the level of the right atrium. These effusions, which complicate cardiac surgery in particular, may compress the right atrium and reduce it to a thin slit.

However, the absence of a pericardial effusion on echocardiography does not rule out the diagnosis of acute pericarditis, which may be accompanied by a small, non-detectable exudation. Finally, a relapsing pericarditis without any recognized cause may reveal a bronchogenic cyst rupture in the pericardium.

As far as the aetiological diagnosis of effusions is concerned, in rare cases echocardiography can give an indication of the nature of the effusion. For

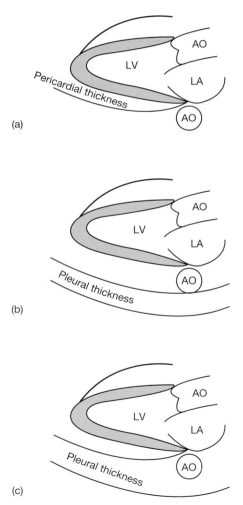

Figure 7.25 Differential diagnosis by location (in the parasternal, long-axis view) between (a) a pericardial effusion and (b) a left pleural effusion. (c) Association of the pericardial and pleural effusions. AO, aorta; LA, left atrium; LV, left ventricle.

example, the visualization of irregular masses in the pericardial sac may indicate a neoplastic origin of the effusion.

Pitfalls when quantifying the size of pericardial effusion

M-mode echocardiography, in the parasternal long-axis view, allows approximate quantification of the size of pericardial effusion (Table 7.9). This semi-quantification is valid if the effusion is uniformly distributed in the pericardial sac. 2D echocardiography appears to be more reliable for evaluating the size of the effusion. Moreover, it allows the precise location of the effusion to be determined, especially in the case of pericardial isolation or localized and isolated separations in unusual locations. 2D echocardiography also makes it possible to confirm the circumferential nature of the effusion. In the presence of a sizeable pericardial effusion, 2D echocardiography shows the dilatation of the oblique pericardial sinus situated behind the left atrium.

A false mitral prolapse and a false SAM may be recorded using M-mode echocardiography; these are artificially created by the cardiac hyperkinesia accompanying a sizeable pericardial effusion. Finally, it should be noted that a small, localized permanent pericardial effusion may persist as a sequela to pericarditis. Its presence should be noted in the report of the echocardiographic examination in order to follow the potential evolution of the pericarditis towards chronicity.

Identification of cardiac tamponade

The diagnosis of cardiac tamponade remains, first and foremost, a clinical diagnosis. Nevertheless, Doppler echocardiography is highly useful for appreciating the poor haemodynamic tolerance of the pericardial effusion. In the presence of a usually large effusion, certain echocardiographic signs suggest cardiac tamponade (Box 7.11). Familiarity with these signs makes it possible to avoid underdiagnosis of cardiac tamponade, which may have grave consequences for the patient. The principal sign of tamponade is compression of the cardiac chambers, essentially the right chambers, due to the increase in intrapericardial pressures (Fig. 7.26). The characteristic appearance of the 'swinging heart' corresponds to an exaggerated swing of the heart inside a pericardial sac of

Table 7.9 Echocardiographic semi-quantification of the pericardial effusion according to its distribution and the size of the epicardial–pericardial dissection measured during diastole

Effusion size	Volume (ml)	Epicardial–pericardial separation
Small	< 300	Purely posterior, < 10 mm
Moderate	300–500	Posterior, 10–20 mm More or less circumferential
Large	> 500	Posterior, > 20 mm Circumferential

Box 7.11   Echocardiographic and Doppler signs of cardiac tamponade

Echocardiographic signs (M-mode, 2D)
- Diastolic compression of the right chambers:
  - early and mid-diastolic collapse of the right ventricle
  - end-diastolic collapse of the right atrium
- Abnormal respiratory variations in the ventricular dimensions:
  - inspiratory enlargement of the RV
  - inspiratory reduction of the LV (the reverse phenomenon is produced in expiration)
- Abnormal cardiac hyperkinesia ('swinging heart' appearance)
- Dilatation of the inferior vena cava, with no reduction in its diameter on inspiration

Doppler signs
- Inspiratory increase in the pulmonary and tricuspid flow velocities
- Inspiratory reduction in the mitral and aortic flow velocities
- Reduction in the aortic ejection time
- Inspiratory lengthening of the LV isovolumic relaxation time
- Disappearance or even inversion of the diastolic flow in the vena cava and subhepatic veins

LV, left ventricle; RV, right ventricle.

---

low mobility. Compression of the left chambers is more rare, and is mainly seen in cases of localized effusion.

Poor tolerance in a pericardial effusion is responsible for major respiratory variation in the intracardiac flow, the equivalent of the clinical paradoxical pulse. In fact, the right ventricular flow increases during inspiration and decreases during expiration: the left ventricular flow undergoes the opposite changes. During tamponade, these respiratory variations are higher than 30% on average, whereas normally these variations do not exceed 15–20%. However, this major respiratory variation in the flows is not specific to tamponade, and may be seen in other circumstances (Box 7.12).

Box 7.12   Causes of major respiratory variations of the right and left intracardiac flows

- Cardiac tamponade
- Chronic constrictive pericarditis
- Chronic obstructive bronchiopathy
- Major tricuspid regurgitation
- Infarction of right ventricle

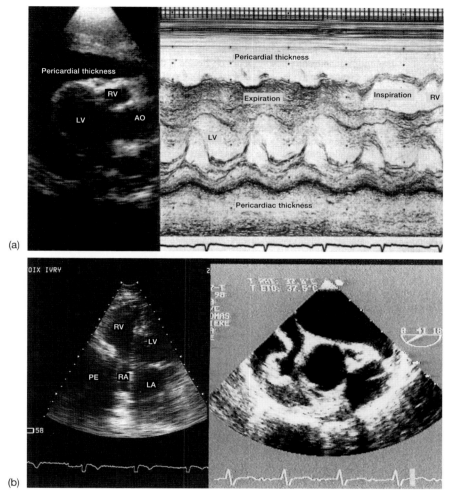

Figure 7.26 Examples of cardiac tamponade. (a) Large pericardial effusion with expiratory compression of the right ventricle and wall hyperkinesia (M-mode). (b) Large pericardial effusion (PE) compressing the right atrium (TTE and TEE). AO, aorta; LA, left atrium; LV, left ventricle; RA, right atrium; RV, right ventricle.

Pitfalls when diagnosing constrictive chronic pericarditis (Fig. 7.27)

Chronic constrictive pericarditis is a difficult clinical entity to diagnose, despite all the available methods of investigation. The condition is characterized by a retractile symphysis of thickened pericardium, which hampers the diastolic distension of the ventricles, and therefore the ventricular filling. It ends in adiastole, the ventricular pressure curve showing the dip–plateau form. The echocardiographic and Doppler signs that may point to a diagnosis of constrictive

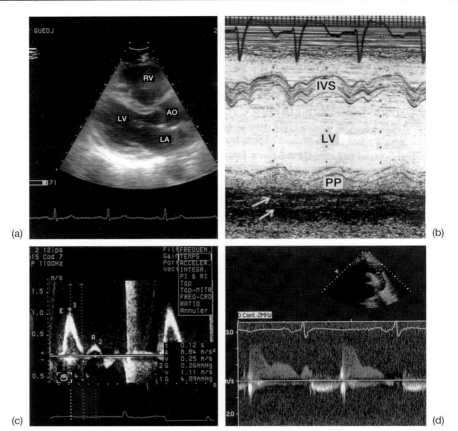

Figure 7.27 Chronic constrictive pericarditis. (a, b) Severe thickening of the pericardium (2D, M-mode); paradoxical septal motion (M-mode). (c, d) Restrictive-type transmitral flow (c); dip–plateau appearance of the pulmonary regurgitant flow. AO, aorta; IVS, interventricular septum; LA, left atrium; LV, left ventricle; RV, right ventricle. (Images by Dr S. Lafitte.)

pericarditis are summarized in Box 7.13. It is important to be familiar with these signs in order to avoid incorrect diagnoses. In fact, the filling of a patient suffering from a pericardial constriction is characterized by both a reduction in left ventricular filling during inspiration, and an expiratory constraint in right ventricular filling. However, the 'restrictive' transmitral flow (E >> A, short deceleration time (DT) and isovolumic relaxation time (IVRT)), reflecting the left adiastole, is not specific to constrictive pericarditis. It may also be observed in other pathological situations leading to elevated left ventricular filling pressures. Moreover, it is influenced by different parameters (age, heart rate, load conditions, conduction disturbance, etc.). The tricuspid flow shows the same changes as the mitral flow in the presence of constriction. The pulmonary venous flow characterized by a reduction in the S wave, and an increase in the

---

Box 7.13   Echocardiographic and Doppler signs of chronic constrictive pericarditis

Echocardiographic signs (M-mode, 2D)
- Abnormal thickening and pericardial rigidity
- Left ventricular filling anomalies:
  - abnormal septal motion (sharp movement towards the LV during early diastole, then recoil during the atrial contraction)
  - abnormal posterior wall motion (rapid posterior movement during early diastole followed by a mid- to end-diastolic horizontalization)
- Other signs:
  - dilatation of the atria, the right ventricle, the inferior vena cava, the subhepatic veins and the pulmonary veins
  - reduction in size of the LV
  - disappearance of the respiratory variations of the inferior vena cava

Doppler signs
- Mitral flow:
  - ↑ E, ↓ A (E >> A), DT < 130 ms, IVRT < 60 ms
  - inspiratory ↓ of the E wave velocities
- Aortic flow:
  - inspiratory reduction in the maximum velocities
- Tricuspid flow:
  - ↑ E, ↓ A, (E >> A), DT < 150 ms
  - Inspiratory ↑ of the E wave velocities
- Pulmonary flow:
  - premature opening of the pulmonary valve
  - modified pulmonary regurgitated diastolic flow (see Table 7.10)
- Pulmonary venous flow:
  - ↓ S (S < D), ↑ A
- Subhepatic venous flow:
  - ↓ S (S < D), ↑ A

DT, deceleration time; IVRT, isovolumic relaxation time; LV, left ventricle.

---

duration and amplitude of the A wave is also influenced by certain parameters (left ventricular compliance and contractility, left atrial relaxation and contractility, flutters, associated major mitral regurgitation, etc.).

As far as the pulmonary regurgitation (PR) flow is concerned, the right adiastole is expressed by three morphological types of PR, reflecting the increasing severity of the constriction (Table 7.10 and Fig. 7.28).

Type III PR shows severe right adiastole: the end-diastolic pressure of the right ventricle is greater than the pressure in the pulmonary artery. However, the interpretation of the PR flow in the context of possible pericardial constriction is difficult in the case of large PR, pulmonary arterial hypertension, tachycardia or flutters.

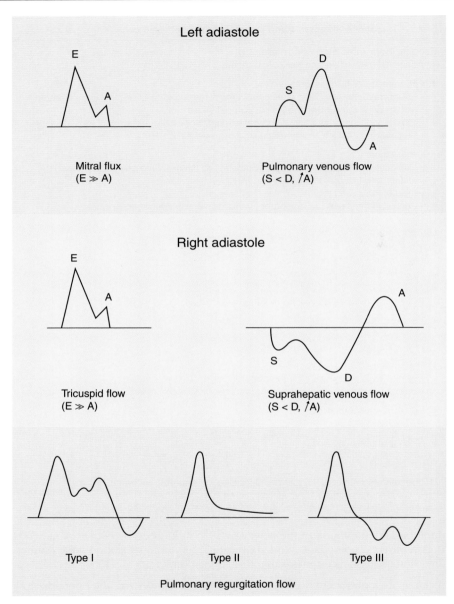

Figure 7.28   Schematic drawing of the Doppler flows reflecting the left adiastole and right adiastole in cases of chronic constrictive pericarditis. Bottom: three types of pulmonary regurgitation.

Table 7.10   Three morphological types of pulmonary regurgitation (PR) in constrictive pericarditis

Type	Characteristics
Type 1 (dip–plateau appearance)	Rapid PR deceleration slope (> 3.7 m/s^{-2}) Short pressure half-time (< 100 ms)
Type II (monophasic appearance)	Sharp cancellation of the PR velocities in mid- to end-diastole
Type III (biphasic appearance)	Retrograde PR flow associated with the anteretrograde presystolic flow

Finally, the flow in the suprahepatic veins is analogous to the pulmonary venous flow (a reduction in the S wave and an increase in the A wave).

DTI applied to the mitral ring may be useful in the diagnosis of a pericardial constriction that is manifested as an annular E wave (Ea) > 8 cm/s and a mitral E/annular E wave (Em/Ea) ratio of < 15. In addition, with DTI it is possible to distinguish between a constrictive pericarditis and a restrictive cardiomyopathy, which is characterized by Ea < 8 cm/s and Em/Ea > 15. The differential echocardiographic diagnosis between these two pathologies is summarized in Table 7.11.

In conclusion, the pitfalls encountered when diagnosing chronic constrictive pericarditis essentially relate to the interpretation of the changes in the ventricular filling profile seen in Doppler echocardiography. A careful analysis of the PR flows enables strong diagnostic arguments to be made in favour of a pericardial constriction.

Table 7.11   Differential echocardiographic diagnosis between chronic constrictive pericarditis and restrictive cardiomyopathy

Parameters	Constrictive pericarditis	Restrictive cardiomyopathy
Size of LV	Reduced	Reduced or normal
Size of RV	Increased	Normal
Biatrial dilation	Yes (+)	Yes (+++)
Left ventricular hypertrophy	No	Yes
Abnormal septal motion	Yes (+++)	Yes (+)
Posterior wall hypokinesia	Yes	Yes
Left ventricular ejection fraction	Normal	Normal or low
Thick pericardium	Yes	No
Pericardial effusion	No or small	Frequent, moderate
Dilated vena cava, low compliance	Yes	Yes
Mitral, tricuspid flows	Restrictive or pseudo-normal	Restrictive
Venous flow: pulmonary subhepatic	$S < D$ A increased	$S < D$ A increased
PR flow	Dip–plateau, PHT < 150 ms	Dip–plateau, PHT < 150 ms
Mitral annular velocity in DTI	Ea > 8 cm/s	Ea < 8 cm/s
Em/Ea ratio	< 15	> 15
Mitral propagation velocity in colour M-mode	Pv > 55 cm/s	Pv < 45 cm/s
Em/Pv ratio	< 2	> 2/5
Inspiratory velocity: mitral E wave (Em) tricuspid E wave	Reduced Increased	Slightly modified Slightly reduced

DTI, Doppler tissue imaging; Ea, annular E wave; Em, mitral E wave; LV, left ventricle; PHT, pressure half-time; PR, pulmonary regurgitation; Pv, propagation velocity; RV, right ventricle.

8

Cardiac chambers

The pitfalls that may be encountered during echocardiographic examination of the cardiac chambers relate to the diagnosis of:

- ventricular and/or atrial dilatation
- intracardiac anatomical structures
- intrachamber masses

PITFALLS RELATING TO CHAMBER DILATATION

Ventricular dilatation

The study of the left ventricle (LV) in M-mode echocardiography requires a high level of recording quality in order to obtain reliable and reproducible results. The causes of errors in the measurement of the internal diameters of the LV using M-mode are:

- poor definition of the endocardium
- an oblique transventricular M-mode projection, which overestimates the ventricular diameters (see Figs 7.2 and 7.3); the technique known as 'anatomical M-mode' is particularly useful in this case (see Fig. 7.4)
- imprecise detection of the end-diastole (diastolic diameter) and/or the end-systole (systolic diameter).

The end-diastole is generally identified as the beginning of the Q wave (American Society of Echocardiography (ASE) technique) or the peak of the R wave of the QRS complex (Pennsylvania (PENN) technique).

At end-systole, the measurements are made using one of two methods:

- at the maximum of the septal movement, when this is normal
- at the maximum of the contraction of the posterior wall, when the septal movement is abnormal.

The internal diameters of the LV are measured according to the approriate convention (Fig. 8.1, and see Fig. 7.1).

Nevertheless, the measurement of the end-systolic diameter of the LV (and thus of the left ventricuar end-systolic surface area (LVSA)) should be abandoned (and consequently also the calculation of the shortening fraction) in the case of paradoxical septal motion.

The normal values of the ventricular diameters in adults are summarized in Table 8.1. However, it is strongly recommended that the patient's size be taken into account in order to interpret the end-diastolic diameter (EDD) of the LV, in particular. A correction of the EDD values for the body surface area is recommended. In practice, the threshold values of 56 mm (absolute values) or 32 mm/m² (as a function of the body surface area) are more often used for EDD. Values above these thresholds confirm dilatation of the LV. However, the dilatation may be non-homogeneous, e.g. an aneurysmal dilatation involving only the apical region of the LV (Fig. 8.2). In fact, the EDD measured classically using M-mode corresponds to the internal diameter of the basal region of the LV only.

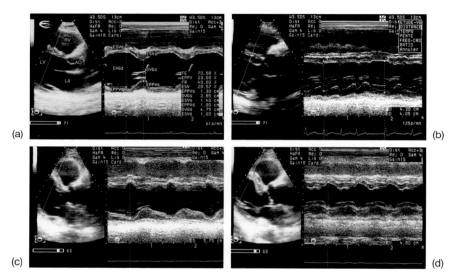

(a)   (b)   (c)   (d)

Figure 8.1   Measurement of the internal diameters of the left ventricle (LV) in 2D M-mode. (a) Correct M-mode projection perpendicular to the ventricular walls. (b) Variations in the diastolic diameter during continuous arrhythmia. (c) Overestimation of the diastolic diameter in the presence of a septal kink, and (d) the corrected diameter obtained using a less oblique projection. AO, aorta; LA, left atrium; RV, right ventricle.

Table 8.1   Normal values in adults of the end-diastolic and end-systolic diameters, and the end-diastolic and end-systolic surfaces of the left ventricle (LV) in transthoracic echocardiography (TTE)

Left ventricular parameter	Values		
	Average	Extreme	Corrected
End-diastolic diameter (EDD)	46 ± 4 mm	38–56 mm	22–32 mm/m²
End-systolic diameter (ESD)	29 ± 3 mm	22–40 mm	15–21 mm/m²
End-diastolic area (LVDA)	32.7 ± 5.8 cm²	21–42 cm²	–
End-systolic surface area (LVSA)	13.9 ± 3.1 cm²	8–19 cm²	–
Body surface area in m².			

A precise two-dimensional (2D) study of the size of the LV is therefore necessary in order to avoid diagnostic errors due to localized ventricular dilatations.

The optimum visualization of the internal contours of the LV, in the apical four-chamber projection, makes it possible to measure the left ventricular end-diastolic surface area (LVDA) and left ventricular end-systolic surface area (LVSA) using the planimetry technique (normal values are summarized in Table 8.1). However, these measures, which deliberately exclude the papillary muscles, are rarely used as a matter of routine, due to their relatively low reliability and reproducibility.

Echocardiographic measurement of the right ventricle (RV) is difficult, due to the complex form of the RV, wrapped around the LV. In practice, the internal diameter of the RV is measured at end-diastole, using M-mode echocardiography in the parasternal, long-axis view. The norm in adults examined in the dorsal decubitus is on average 13.6 ± 2.6 mm, with values ranging between 7 mm and 23 mm. In the left lateral decubitus, the diameter of the normal RV is slightly increased (9–26 mm). Moreover, the diameter of the RV may vary in a physiological manner with respiration (an increase on inspiration of 2–3 mm). Due to the high individual variability of the right ventricular diameter, it is preferable to use the ratio of the left and right ventricular diameters during diastole (RV/LV), which is normally around 0.33.

The diameters of the LV and RV may also be measured using 2D echocardiography (Fig. 8.3).

Dilatation of the atria
Echocardiography can be used to evaluate the diameters and the surface area of the left atrium (LA). The anteroposterior diameter of the LA is routinely

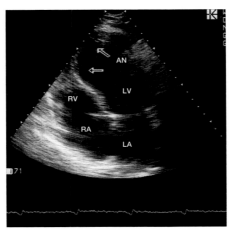

Figure 8.2   Non-homogeneous dilatation of the left ventricle (LV): voluminous aneurysm (AN) of the septoapical region of an infarcted LV (arrows). LA, left atrium; RA, right atrium; RV, right ventricle.

Diastole

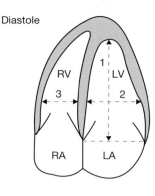

Systole

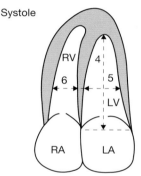

		Extreme values (mm)	Average value (mm)
Diastole	1	73–90	79 ± 4
	2	34–56	42 ± 5
	3	30–41	33 ± 6
Systole	4	48–69	58 ± 5
	5	25–41	30 ± 5
	6	21–37	23 ± 6

Figure 8.3 Normal values in adults for the left and right ventricular diameters in transthoracic 2D echocardiography. Measurements carried out according to the four-chamber projection during diastole and systole. AO, aorta; LA, left atrium; LV, left ventricle; RA, right atrium; RV, right ventricle.

measured in M-mode using the parasternal, long-axis view during end-diastole (Fig. 8.4). This is a simple measurement, and its accuracy is usually good. The potential limitations concerning the measurement of the anteroposterior diameter of the LA are:

- an oblique M-mode projection, which overestimates the diameter (Fig. 8.5)
- the sometimes poor definition of the posterior endocardium of the LA
- an asymmetric dilatation of the LA.

In fact, measuring only the anteroposterior diameter in the long-axis projection is insufficient in the case of asymmetrical enlargement or non-homogeneous dilatation of the LA, which is frequently observed in older patients. In these situations, it is recommended that the superoinferior diameter of the LA is also measured. This diameter is measured using the 2D mode (apical cross-section of the four chambers) from the plane of the mitral annulus to the base of the LA, during systole (Figs 8.4 and 8.6). The normal values for these two atrial diameters as measured using echocardiography are summarized in Table 8.2.

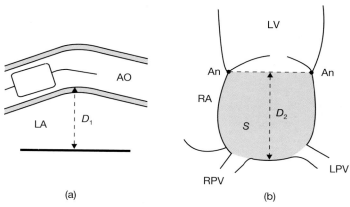

Figure 8.4 Measurements of the left atrium: (a) in M-mode echocardiography, anteroposterior diameter (D_1); (b) in 2D echocardiography, apical four-chamber view, superoinferior diameter (D_2), surface area (S) measured by planimetry. An, plane of mitral annulus; AO, aorta; LA, left atrium; LPV, left pulmonary vein; LV, left ventricle; RA, right atrium; RPV, right pulmonary vein.

Table 8.2   Normal values of the LA diameters and surface area in adults as measured using TTE during systole

Diameter	Value	
	Average	Extremes
Anteroposterior (M-mode)	30 ± 3 mm (16 mm/m²)	23–38 mm (12–22 mm/m²)
Superoinferior (2D)	41 ± 6 mm	29–43 mm
Surface (2D)	14.8 ± 2.1 cm²	13.6–16.8 cm²

In practice, in order to confirm the dilatation of the LA, its size must be measured in at least two projections: parasternal and apical (see Fig. 8.2). The threshold values of 40 mm for the anteroposterior diameter and 45 mm for the superoinferior diameter are generally retained. In order to confirm the diagnosis of dilatation of the LA, it is useful also to measure the surface area of the atrium. This measurement is made during systole, using planimetry and the apical four-chamber projection (see Fig. 8.4). This gives the maximum end-systolic surface area of the LA. The LA is considered to be dilated if the surface area measured with planimetry exceeds 15 cm² (see Fig. 8.6).

The limitations of the planimetric method are:

- poorly visualized internal contours of the LA
- off-axis projections, which may over- or underestimate the actual surface area of the LA
- poor definition of the plane of the mitral annulus (the 'floor' of the LA) or the junction of the pulmonary veins (the 'roof' of the LA).

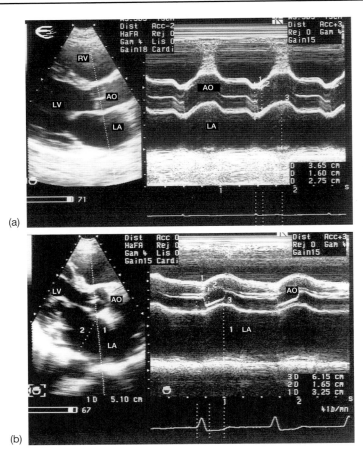

Figure 8.5 Measurement of the anteroposterior diameter of the left atrium (LA) using M-mode in the parasternal, long-axis projection. (a) Correct measurement, made perpendicular to the walls.(b) Oblique M-mode projection, increasing the measured diameter of the LA to 61 mm (actual diameter in 2D is 51 mm). AO, aorta; LV, left ventricle; RV, right ventricle.

A surface area of the right atrium (RA), also measured using planimetry in the apical four-chamber projection, of > 14 cm^2 suggests that it is dilated (Fig. 8.7). The echocardiographic measurement of the diameter of the RA is not precise, and therefore contributes little information.

Dilatation of the left atrial appendage

The left atrial appendage (LAA) is practically unexplorable using transthoracic echocardiography (TTE). In contrast, transoesophageal echocardiography (TEE), particularly in the multiplanar mode, allows visualization of the LAA, which is seen as a horn-shaped area separated from the left upper pulmonary vein by an anatomical fold that is seen in the shape of a club. Planimetry can be used to measure the surface area of the LAA, and flow through the LAA can be

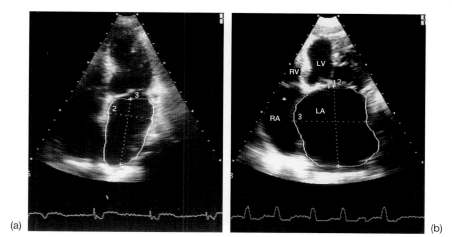

Figure 8.6 Non-homogeneous dilatation of the left atrium (LA). (a) Normal anteroseptal diameter (38 mm), increased superoinferior diameter (59 mm). Surface area of the LA measured using planimetry = 20 cm². (b) Ectasic dilatation of the LA: anteroposterior diameter = 63 mm, superoinferior diameter = 71 mm; surface area measured using planimetry = 41 cm². LV, left ventricle; RA, right atrium; RV, right ventricle.

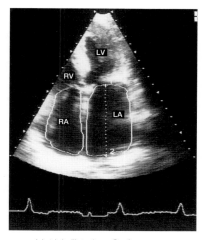

Figure 8.7 Non-homogeneous biatrial dilatation. Surface area measured using planimetry: left atrium (LA) 32 cm², right atrium (RA) 22 cm². LV, left ventricle; RV, right ventricle.

studied using Doppler TEE. Typically, normal flow through the LAA shows a quadriphasic pattern, with a positive phase due to emptying of the LAA followed by an inversion of the flow corresponding to filling of the LAA. Normally, the surface area of the LAA is less than 6 cm² (in transverse cross-section) and the LAA emptying velocity is generally > 50 cm/s (Fig. 8.8). Finally, the right atrial appendage is rarely identifiable using TEE (Fig. 8.9).

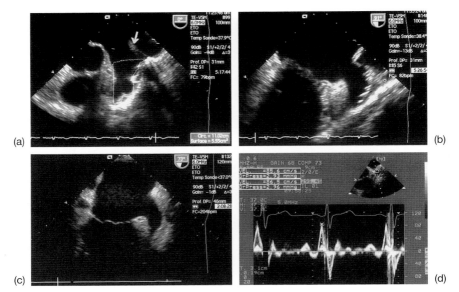

Figure 8.8   Study of the left atrial appendage (LAA) using TEE. Different morphological appearances of the LAA: (a) normal (surface area 5.5 cm²), with anatomical fold (arrow); (b) trabeculated; (c) without fold. (d) Normal LAA flow, with emptying and filling velocities close to 86 cm/s.

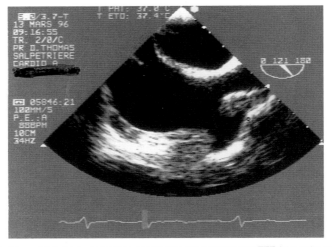

Figure 8.9   Normal left atrial appendage visualized using multiplanar TEE (triangular appearance).

Echocardiographic pitfalls relating to investigating the LAA are generally due to:

- the technical difficulties associated with optimum visualization of the LAA
- unusual forms of the LAA (non-triangular shape or without fold) (see Fig. 8.8(c))

Table 8.3   Threshold values used in practice to diagnose chamber dilatation when using TTE

Structure	Measure	Value
Left ventricle	End-diastolic diameter	> 56 mm, > 32 mm/m²
	End-diastolic surface area	> 42 cm²
Right ventricle	End-diastolic diameter	> 25 mm, > 15 mm/m²
	End-diastolic surface area	> 22 cm²
Left atrium	Anteroposterior diameter	> 40 mm
	Superoinferior diameter	> 45 mm
	Maximum surface area	> 15 cm²
Right atrium	Anteroposterior diameter	> 37 mm
	Superoinferior diameter	> 42 mm
	Maximum surface area	> 14 cm²
Left atrial appendage	Maximum surface area	> 6 cm²

- numerous trabeculations of the bottom of the auricle due to the pectinated muscles, which may simulate a thrombus in the appendage (see Fig. 8.8(b))
- planimetry errors: the normal LAA surface area measured in the transverse cross-section (at 0° in multiplanar TEE) is higher (4.5 ± 1.1 cm²) than that measured in the longitudinal cross-section (at 90°) (3.6 ± 1.2 cm²)
- incomplete recordings of the LAA flow, which may lead to incorrect interpretation of the image obtained.

Finally, the LAA may be invisible in TEE due to ligation or surgical resection.

PITFALLS RELATING TO INTRACARDIAC CHAMBER STRUCTURES

Excluding congenital cardiopathies from the discussion, the 'anatomical' pitfalls that may be encountered during echocardiographic examination (TTE and/or TEE) are due to physiological or pathological intracardiac structures. Familiarity with these structures is necessary in order to avoid diagnostic errors.

Physiological structures (Box 8.1)

The physiological structures that may be found in the cardiac chambers are:

- Numerous trabeculations of the walls of the RV, suggesting a hypertrophic cardiomyopathy.
- Structures identifiable in the RA:
  - the Eustachian valve, the entry valve of the orifice of the inferior vena cava (IVC), prolapsing by 1 or 2 cm into the RA (Fig. 8.10), is membranous in appearance and may vary in size

---

Box 8.1   Physiological anatomical structures of the heart identifiable using echocardiography

- Right ventricular trabeculations
- Right intra-atrial structures:
  - the Eustachian valve
  - the Chiari network
  - the crista terminalis
- Left chamber structures:
  - the coronary sinus
  - the oblique pericardial sinus
  - 'physiological' mitral valvular ballooning

- the Chiari network, an embryological structure of thin threads situated between the IVC and the interatrial septum, appears as a floating net
- the crista terminalis, the muscular spur situated at the level of the lateral wall of the RA.
- Structures relating to the left chambers:
  - the coronary sinus, which is situated at the atrioventricular junction
  - the oblique pericardial sinus, which is located behind the LA
  - physiological ballooning of the mitral valve (an anatomical variant of the normal mitral valve), which is seen in children and younger subjects.

The coronary and pericardial sinuses may mimic a localized pericardial effusion when dilated (see page 130).

Pathological structures

So-called 'abnormal' pathological anatomical structures that may be detected using echocardiography are summarized in Box 8.2. Structures of this type may also constitute a source of false echocardiographic diagnoses (Figs 8.10 and 8.11).

Box 8.2   Pathological anatomical structures of the heart identifiable using echocardiography

- Left intraventricular false tendons (transversal or longitudinal types) (see page 99)
- Moderator band of the right ventricle (see page 99)
- Coarse trabeculations of the right ventricle
- Septal kinking (see page 103)
- Subaortic septal rim (see page 99)
- Atrial septal aneurysm
- Patent foramen ovale discovered accidentally in apparently healthy subjects
- Fibrin strands attached to the native valves or the pulmonary veins

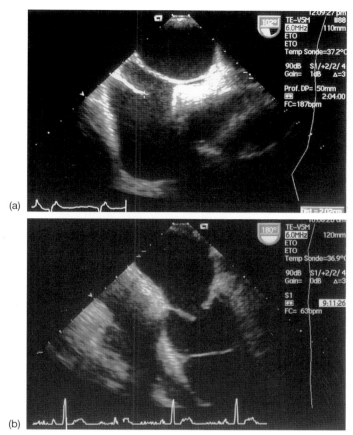

Figure 8.10   Intracardiac anatomical structures seen in TEE: (a) Eustachian valve; (b) intra-left ventricular transverse false tendon.

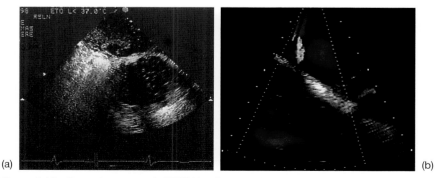

Figure 8.11   Patent foramen ovale (PFO) identified using TEE and the contrast test: (a) passage of contrast from the right to the left atrium through the PFO; (b) interatrial shunt flow traversing the PFO as seen in 2D colour Doppler.

PITFALLS RELATING TO INTRACARDIAC MASSES

With the help of echocardiography, especially TEE, it is possible to visualize abnormal intrachamber masses such as:

- thrombi with or without spontaneous contrast (Fig. 8.12)
- endocardial vegetations (see Figs 6.37 and 6.38)
- intracardiac tumours (Fig. 8.13)
- massive valvular or annular calcifications
- marked myxomatous degeneration of the valves.

The diagnosis of these intracardiac masses is based on 2D echocardiography. The common echocardiographic pitfalls relating to this diagnosis are summarized in Box 8.3. A thrombus of the LA, and in particular of the LAA, is often associated with a spontaneous contrast reflecting a prethrombotic state. This spontaneous contrast, corresponding to a blood stasis, appears on 2D imaging in the form of mobile echoes circulating in 'wisps of smoke' (Fig. 8.14). It is vital to adjust the reception gains of the machine correctly in order to clearly show the spontaneous contrast. A positive diagnosis of spontaneous contrast requires low gain values, especially in cases of concentrated micro echoes. In practical terms, there is a distinction between:

- intense spontaneous contrast, where the entire LA is filled with scattered echoes visible at low gain
- slight spontaneous contrast, where only part of the LA contains scattered echoes visible at high gain.

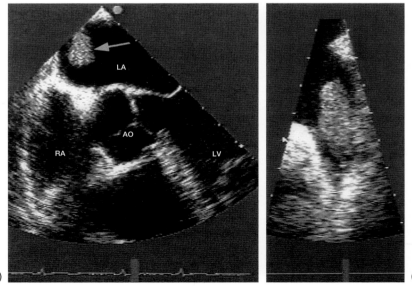

(a)　　　　　　　　　　　　　　　　　　　　　　　　　　　　(b)

Figure 8.12　Examples of thrombi identified using TEE: (a) in the left atrium (LA); (b) in the left atrial appendage. AO, aorta; LV, left ventricle; RA, right atrium.

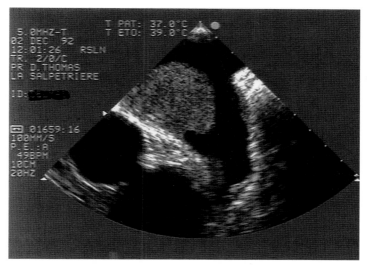

Figure 8.13 Myxoma of the left atrium visualized using TEE.

Box 8.3   Echocardiographic pitfalls relating to the detection of an abnormal intrachamber mass

Technical pitfalls
- Patient hypoechogenicity leading to false-negative diagnoses
- Ultrasound artefacts (reverberations from a denser structure)
- Poor adjustment of the machine (i.e. settings)
- Failure to use multiple echocardiographic projections

Diagnostic pitfalls
- Small volume of the mass (< 3 mm), preventing its echocardiographic identification
- Low echogenicity of the mass, limiting its detection (e.g. recent thrombus)
- Atypical location of the mass (e.g. myxoma located in the right ventricle)
- Mass adhering to the cardiac wall (mural thrombus, tumour infiltrating the myocardium, etc.)
- Regression or disappearance of the mass in certain situations (e.g. treated or migrating thrombus)
- Differential diagnosis between:
  - calcified, organized, aged thrombi and nodular valvular calcifications
  - valvular vegetations and a localized myxomatous valvular degeneration
- Incorrect interpretation of cardiac structures (muscular trabeculations, large papillary muscle, left atrial folds, etc.) leading to false-positive diagnoses
- Neglect of the clinical context, which can direct the echocardiographic diagnosis

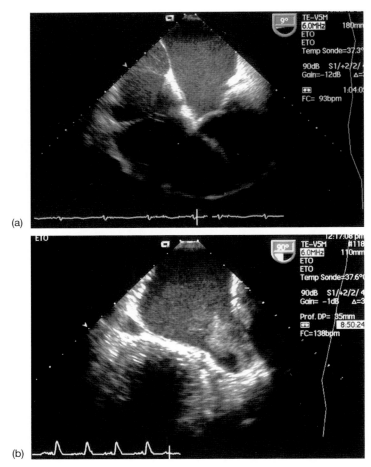

Figure 8.14   Spontaneous contrast detected using TEE: (a) intense in the left atrium (LA); (b) massive and turbulent in the LA and the left atrial appendage.

The spontaneous contrast should be searched for thoroughly using echocardiography, especially TEE, in the pathological situations summarized in Box 8.4.

Finally, artificial structures (such as valvular or vascular prostheses, pacing wires, intracardiac catheters, etc.) may be visualized in echocardiography (Fig. 8.15).

Box 8.4   Pathological situations responsible for the formation of a spontaneous contrast

- Mitral valvulopathies: valvular stenoses, severe decompensated mitral regurgitation
- Following mitral valve replacement
- Severe dilated cardiomyopathy
- Ectasia or post-infarction left ventricular aneurysm
- Aortic dissection (spontaneous contrast in the false lumen)
- Low cardiac output (intra-aortic spontaneous contrast)
- Atrial fibrillation with a dilated left atrium
- Constrictive pericarditis (spontaneous contrast in the inferior vena cava)
- Cardiac grafts

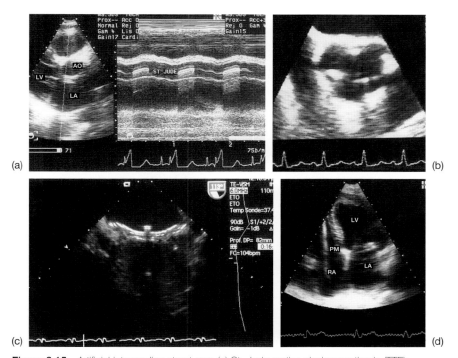

Figure 8.15   Artificial intracardiac structures: (a) St. Jude aortic valvular prosthesis (TTE); (b) aortic bioprosthesis (TEE); (c) atrial trans-septal prosthesis (Amplatzer Septal Occluder) (TEE); (d) right intrachamber cardiac pacemaker (PM) (TTE). AO, aorta; LA, left atrium; LV, left ventricle; RA, right atrium.

9

Systolic and diastolic function of the ventricles

The pitfalls of Doppler echocardiography when evaluating the systolic and diastolic function of the heart are discussed separately for the left and the right ventricles.

PITFALLS WHEN EVALUATING THE SYSTOLIC AND DIASTOLIC FUNCTION OF THE LEFT VENTRICLE

Doppler echocardiography has assumed a leading and irreplaceable role in the evaluation of left ventricular function. Various parameters for assessing the function of the left ventricle (LV) have been proposed, but none is formally discriminative. Moreover, Doppler echocardiography remains an operator-dependent technique with many limitations. Nevertheless, this modality does make it possible to separate systolic and diastolic dysfunction of the LV, which differ both in their prognosis and in their treatment.

Evaluation of the systolic function of the left ventricle
Among the echo Doppler parameters that can be used to evaluate the systolic function of the LV, the most commonly used remain the shortening fraction and the ejection fraction, to which may sometimes be added the cardiac output (Box 9.1).

Systolic shortening fraction of the left ventricle
The systolic shortening fraction (SF) roughly corresponds to the pumping function of the LV, resting on the following hypothesis: the shortening of the

---

Box 9.1   Usual echo Doppler parameters used in the analysis of the systolic and diastolic left ventricular function

Systolic parameters
- Systolic shortening fraction
- Ejection fraction
- Aortic output

Diastolic parameters
- Mitral flow profile
- Left ventricular isovolumic relaxation time
- Pulmonary venous flow profile
- Propagation velocity of the mitral flow
- Displacement velocity of the mitral flow

minor axis of the LV is a reflection of the overall systolic function. In practice, this is a simple parameter to calculate. It is well correlated with the angiographic ejection fraction and is used almost systematically (Fig. 9.1). The SF is derived from the M-mode measurement of the diameters of the LV at end-diastole (EDD) and in end-systole (ESD):

SF = EDD – ESD/EDD

The normal value of the SF is 36 ± 6%. This parameter is, however, not ideal, because it is derived from a measurement made at only one level of the ventricle. In fact, the SF explores only the basal part of the LV and does not take

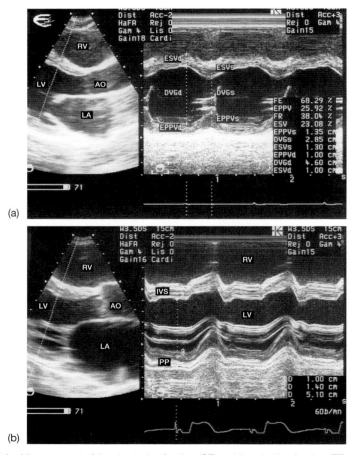

(a)

(b)

Figure 9.1   Measurement of the shortening fraction (SF) and the ejection fraction (EF) of the left ventricle (LV) using M-mode. (a) The method is feasible and reliable in the case of homogeneous regional wall motion (SF = 38%; EF = 68%). (b) Measurement of the SF is not possible, because the method is invalid when there is paradoxical septal motion. AO, aorta; IVS, interventricular septum; LA, left atrium; RV, right ventricle.

into account the movement of the other ventricular segments. Thus it is possible to evaluate the overall systolic function of the LV only if its wall motion is homogeneous. The pitfalls of using the SF calculation are summarized in Box 9.2 (see also Fig. 9.1). Moreover, the interpretation of the SF values obtained is sometimes delicate. The SF depends not only on the intrinsic contractility of the LV, but also on the load conditions. Thus, an acute increase in the preload and/or a reduction in the afterload (hypotension, mitral regurgitation, etc.) leads to an increase in the SF. Conversely, an acute decrease in the preload and/or an acute increase in the afterload (e.g. tension pulse) reduces the SF.

Left ventricular ejection fraction

The ejection fraction (EF) is calculated using the end-diastolic volume (EDV) and end-systolic volume (ESV) of the LV as follows:

$$EF = EDV - ESV/EDV$$

The normal value of the EF is $63 \pm 6\%$.

The ventricular volumes may be calculated in one of two ways:

- according to the cube formula (volume $= D^3$) or the Teicholz formula (volume $= 7D^3/2.4 + D$), where D is the ventricular diameter measured using M-mode echocardiography
- using different mathematical models in two-dimensional (2D) echocardiography.

In practice, software integrated into the ultrasound machine allows automatic calculation of the EF according to the volumetric method selected. The EF best expresses the pumping function of the LV. It is nonetheless subject to the same errors as the evaluation of ventricular volumes (Box 9.3). In fact, the cube formula, which is based on the assimilation of the LV into a rotational ellipsoid, the major axis of which is double the minor axis, often overestimates the volumes in the case of left ventricular dilatation. When the LV is dilated, the

---

Box 9.2   Pitfalls relating to the calculation of the left ventricular shortening fraction (SF) using M-mode echocardiography

Failure to respect the calculation conditions:
- Homogeneous wall motion
- Normal ventricular geometry
- M-mode projection perpendicular to the ventricular walls
- Absence of: regional asynergy, complete left bundle branch block, Wolf–Parkinson–White syndrome, paradoxical septal motion, left–right shunt

Dependence of the SF on the following factors:
- Heart rate
- Preload and afterload
- Myocardial contractility

ratio of the major axis to the minor axis decreases and is no longer equal to 2. The Teicholz formula brings a correction factor to the cube formula for the dilated or spherical LV. Whichever formula is used, the calculation is only reliable if the overall contraction of the LV is homogeneous. Obviously, the ventricular diameter as measured obliquely in M-mode, and therefore overestimated, leads inevitably to an overestimation of volume. These numerous restrictions have led to the increasingly frequent use of 2D echocardiography in daily practice to determine the ventricular volumes. Several geometric models have been proposed, on which the calculation of the volumes have been based (monoplanar or biplanar ellipsoid, disc methods, hemi-ellipse/cylinder methods, etc.). Using these different models, the estimation of the volumes is extrapolated on the basis of the ventricular surface areas measured during systole and diastole using planimetry, and of the ventricular dimensions, over one or more 2D cross-sections, according to the model applied (Fig. 9.2).

The quantification of ventricular volumes using 2D echocardiography is more precise than that done using M-mode. The 2D modality is particularly useful and advantageous in cases of deformation of the LV (e.g. aneurysm). It is also valuable in cases of regional wall motion abnormalities; this is often the case in ischaemic cardiopathy. The modality is sufficiently reproducible and reliable when used by a trained operator. However, the 2D method is not exempt from criticism and there are pitfalls in its current use that must be clearly understood (see Box 9.3).

Box 9.3   Pitfalls in the calculation of the left ventricular (LV) ejection fraction (EF) using M-mode and 2D echocardiography

Pitfalls of M-mode echocardiography
- Errors in the measurement of the ventricular diameters
- Overestimation of the volumes using the cube method, in the case of LV dilatation
- Inaccurate calculation of the EF in the case of regional anomalies
- EF calculation invalid in the case of LV deformation (aneurysm, asymmetrical hypertrophy, etc.)

Pitfalls of 2D echocardiography
- Poor quality of the 2D imaging
- Insufficient definition of the endocardium
- Imprecise ventricular measurements (surface area, diameter)
- Inappropriate selection of the method of caculating the volumes
- Frequent underestimation of volumes in 2D
- Poor reproducibility of results by an untrained operator

Pitfalls of M-mode and 2D echocardiography
- Dependence of the EF on afterload conditions
- Failure to take the average of at least three volume measurements

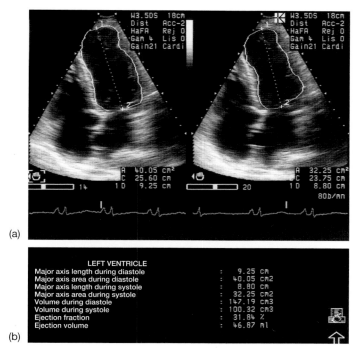

(a)

(b)

LEFT VENTRICLE	
Major axis length during diastole	: 9.25 cm
Major axis area during diastole	: 40.05 cm2
Major axis length during systole	: 8.80 cm
Major axis area during systole	: 32.25 cm2
Volume during diastole	: 147.19 cm3
Volume during systole	: 100.32 cm3
Ejection fraction	: 31.84 %
Ejection volume	: 46.87 ml

Figure 9.2   Calculation of the left ventricular (LV) ejection fraction (EF) using the ventricular volumes measured in the 2D mode according to the 'ellipsoid monoplane' model: (a) 2D apical image of the four chambers frozen in end-diastole and in end-systole; (b) LV systolic dysfunction (EF = 32%).

The routine use of echocardiography shows the difficulty of optimal visualization of the endocardial contours of the LV. This is why it is so important to adjust and use the ultrasound machine correctly, and to select the most echogenic projection, and therefore the most appropriate method deriving from it. Taking an average of at least three measurements is also vital. It is also necessary to exercise prudence in the interpretation of the results, in order to avoid making an arbitrary judgement.

In fact, the left ventricular EF is highly sensitive to variations in the afterload. It is therefore necessary to interpret this parameter in the light of possible modifications in the afterload conditions (increased, as in aortic stenosis or arterial hypertension, or reduced, as in mitral regurgitation).

Technological advances in ultrasound imaging (harmonic imaging; colour kinesis, based on the automatic detection of the contours of the endocardium; myocardial contrast echocardiography) have made possible considerable improvements in the definition of the endocardial contours during systole and diastole, and consequently in the calculation of ventricular volumes in the 2D mode. In parallel, the reproducibility of the examination has been strengthened as a result of these new techniques. Three-dimensional echocardiography also gives access to the measurement of the left ventricular volumes and EF.

Cardiac output

Cardiac Doppler makes it possible to calculate the cardiac output at the level of the four cardiac valves. The calculation of the aortic output (left ventricular outflow) is the simplest and most commonly used method in current practice. The aortic output (Q_{AO}) may be considered as a reflection of the systolic performance of the LV. It is calculated by using echo Doppler at the subaortic level, and then multiplying the subaortic velocity–time integral (VTI) by the surface area of the outflow chamber of the LV (S) and the heart rate (HR):

$$Q_{AO} = VTI \times S \times HR$$

To calculate the left ventricular outflow tract area, it is sufficient to measure the subaortic diameter (D) using 2D echocardiography and the parasternal, long-axis view (Fig. 9.3):

$$S = \pi D^2/4$$

In a healthy subject, the normal value of the aortic output is in the range 4–7 l/min. The Q_{AO} is generally corrected using the body surface area in order to determine the cardiac index. The cardiac index is considered pathological if its value is < 2.5 l/min/m².

The pitfalls of evaluating the aortic output using the echo Doppler modality are summarized in Box 9.4. They are linked in particular to:

- the assumptions within the output calculation
- a failure to observe the measurement conditions
- errors in the echo Doppler measurement
- an incorrect interpretation of the results.

In fact, the calculation of Q_{AO} in echo Doppler is based on the following assumptions:

- the presence of the laminar aortic flow
- a fixed and circular aortic area
- perfect alignment of the Doppler beam with the aortic flow.

Therefore, for the calculation of the output to be reliable, the subaortic flows should be laminar and flat. This is by no means the case when there is a rim or septal kinking. In the case of a turbulent flow with a parabolic velocity profile (higher velocity at the centre of the orifice) the calculation of the aortic output by this method should be abandoned, rather than be used to calculate a false value.

Poor alignment with the aortic flow leads to underestimation of the subaortic velocity (VTI), and therefore of the aortic output. Thus it is necessary to increase the number of projections explored by varying the site of the Doppler region of interest below the aortic orifice. It is important to note that the subaortic VTI also varies according to the heart rate (Fig. 9.4). Thus, for a given aortic surface area and a given heart rate, the VTI increases as the heart rate decreases, and vice versa.

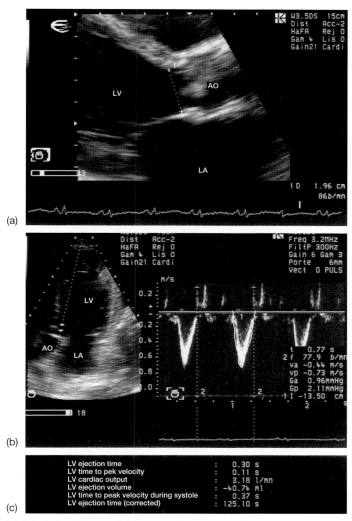

Figure 9.3 Calculation of the cardiac output using the echo Doppler mode. (a) Measurement of the subaortic diameter in the longitudinal, parasternal cross-section, in zoom (D = 1.96 cm). (b) Planimetry of the subaortic flow recorded using pulsed Doppler in the apical cross-section (velocity–time integral (VTI) = 13.5 cm, heart rate = 78 beats/min). (c) Aortic output: $Q_{AO} = 3.14(D/2)^2 \times VTI \times HR = 3.14(1.96)^2 \times 13.5 \times 78 = 3.18$ l/min. AO, aorta; LA, left atrium; LV, left ventricle.

It is important to consider the basic measurements (VTI, D, HR) in order to determine the LV stroke voume precisely, reliably and reproducibly. It must be emphasized that all the measurements used to calculate the output (VTI, D, HR) are interdependent, and that an error in any one of them will produce an

Box 9.4   Pitfalls relating to the calculation of the aortic output using Doppler echocardiography

- Failure to observe the measurement conditions
- Errors in measurement (diameter, velocity–time integral (VTI))
- Variations in the VTI according to the heart rate
- Failure to repeat the measurements (at least three measurements)
- Turbulent valvular flow
- Parabolic blood velocity profile
- Elliptical shape of the valve orifice
- Variations in the surface area of the orifice over the cardiac cycle
- Multiplicity of factors determining the cardiac output
- Uncritical or mistaken interpretation of the result

incorrect result. Therefore, even the smallest of errors (2 mm) in the measurement of the subaortic diameter leads to significant variations in the calculated result; hence the importance of the quality of the 2D image. Finally, the interpretation of Doppler measurements of the aortic output is also complex. The multiple determinants of the cardiac output must be taken into account. Thus, the cardiac output is not an isolated value and should be compared with other clinical (blood pressure, thyroid function, etc.), haemodynamic (venous pressure, capillary pressure, etc.) and echocardiographic (ejection fraction, left ventricular dimensions, associated valvular regurgitation, etc.) data (Table 9.1). Cardiac failure at high cardiac output may point to hypothyroidism, anaemia or an arteriovenous fistula.

As for the measurement of the output at the level of the mitral and tricuspid orifices, the measurement of the aortic output runs into major technical difficulties (elliptical shape of the orifices, continuous variation in the valve surface

Table 9.1   Some examples of haemodynamic profiles in Doppler echocardiography

Condition	Ejection fraction (EF)	Cardiac output (CO)	Left ventricular end-diastolic diameter (EDD)
Normal	Normal	Normal	Normal
Compensated heart failure	Reduced	Normal	Increased
Uncompensated heart failure	Reduced	Reduced	Increased
Hypovolaemia	Increased	Reduced	Normal
Hyperthyroidism	Increased	Increased	Normal

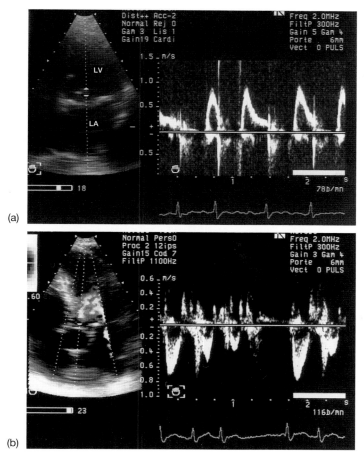

Figure 9.4 Influence of continuous arrhythmia due to atrial fibrillation on the mitral and aortic flow: (a) disappearance of the A wave of the mitral flow; (b) variability in the velocity–time integral of the aortic flow. LA, left atrium; LV, left ventricle.

area during diastole, non-flat velocity profile), rendering this complex measurement less reliable and more difficult to achieve in current practice.

Evaluation of the diastolic function of the left ventricle

The evaluation of the filling of the LV, known as the diastolic function, is one of the cardiologist's daily tasks. The principal parameters of the diastolic function that can be measured using Doppler echocardiography are summarized in Box 9.1. In practice it is more complex to calculate the diastolic function of the LV, which is determined by its relaxation and compliance, than the systolic function of the LV. It is therefore desirable to critically compare the different parameters in order to reliably asess the patient's diastolic function. Precise analysis of the left ventricular filling allows the diagnosis of diastolic cardiac failure, which may be pure, with a conserved ejection fraction, or associated with a systolic dysfunction of the LV. The pitfalls that arise when determining the LV diastolic function using Doppler echocardiography relate to:

- the recording of the Doppler parameters and their interpretation
- the possible presence of a pseudo-normal profile of the mitral flow
- the estimation of the filling pressures of the LV.

Recording and interpretation of diastolic Doppler parameters

Detailed analysis of the Doppler parameters discussed below makes it possible to classify patients into three haemodynamic profiles corresponding to stages of increasing severity of the diastolic dysfunction of the LV (Table 9.2):

- Profile I: abnormal relaxation of the LV
- Profile II: pseudonormal appearance (intermediate stage between profiles I and III)
- Profile III: compliance disturbance of the LV (restrictive profile).

It should be noted that the evolution from one profile of the left ventricular diastolic dysfunction to another is possible in the same patient upon progression of their condition, upon variations in the load conditions, or upon acute haemodynamic modifications or a treatment.

Mitral flow

The mitral flow is recorded using pulsed Doppler at the tip of the funnel formed by the mitral valves. The normal mitral flow comprises an early diastolic E wave of rapid filling of the LV and an end-diastolic A wave due to the atrial contraction (Fig. 9.5).

In practice, the following parameters are measured:

- the E/A ratio (= 1–2)
- the deceleration time (DT) of the E wave, enabling the balancing of the ventricular and atrial pressures (= 150–220 ms)
- the duration of the mitral A wave (MAd) is greater than the duration of the A wave of the pulmonary atrial reversal (PAd) (MAd > PAd).

Classically, these parameters serve to define the left ventricular filling profile (see Table 9.2). The pitfalls encountered in evaluating the diastolic mitral flow in this context are summarized in Box 9.5.

In reality, evaluation of the diastolic mitral flow is complex, as the mitral parameters are highly dependent on the instantaneous pressure gradient between the left atrium and the LV during diastole. In fact, several factors may modify the appearance of the mitral flow (Table 9.3). The left ventricular filling pressures are an essential determining element of the appearance of the mitral flow. Therefore, any reduction in the preload leads to a reduction in the E wave velocity and the E/A ratio, and therefore modifies the appearance towards profile I (abnormal relaxation). Conversely, an increase in the preload (increased pressure in the left atrium) entails a transition towards profile III (impaired

Table 9.2   Characteristics of the three diastolic dysfunction profiles of the left ventricle (LV)

	PROFILE I (abnormal relaxation)	PROFILE II (pseudonormal)	PROFILE III (restrictive)
Mitral flow	• E/A < 1 • DT > 220 ms • IVRT > 100 ms	• E/A • DT normal • IVRT	• E/A >2 • DT < 150 ms • IVRT < 100 ms
Pulmonary venous flow	• S/D > 1 • Normal LV EDP: PA < 35 cm/s PAd < MAd • High LV EDP: PA > 35 cm/s PAd > MAd	• S/D < 1 • PA > 35 cm/s • PAd > MAd	• S/D << 1 • PA > 35 cm/s • PAd > MAd
Colour M-mode	• Pv < 45 cm/s	• Pv < 45 cm/s	• Pv << 45 cm/s
Mitral Doppler tissue imaging	• Ea < 8 cm/s • Ea/Aa < 1	• Ea < 8 cm/s • Ea/Aa < 1	• Ea << 8 cm/s • Ea/Aa > 1

A, A wave; Aa, annular A wave; D, D wave; DT, deceleration time; E, E wave; Ea, annular E wave; IVRT, isovolumic relaxation time; LV EDP, left ventricular end-diastolic pressure; PA, amplitude of the A wave; PAd, duration of A wave of pulmonary venous flow; Pv, propagation velocity; S, S wave; Sa, annular S wave.

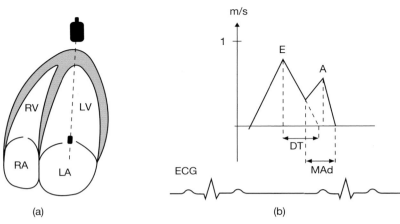

Figure 9.5 Echo Doppler examination of normal mitral flow. (a) Doppler sample volume at the tip of the mitral valve (apical four-chamber view). (b) Schematic appearance of the mitral flow recorded using pulsed Doppler. Measurements: maximum velocities of the E and A waves, deceleration time (DT) of the E wave; mitral A wave duration (MAd). ECG, electrocardiogram; LA, left atrium; LV, left ventricle; RA, right atrium; RV, right ventricle.

compliance). The patient's age has a significant influence on the parameters of the mitral flow (Fig. 9.6). In young or athletic patients, a pseudorestrictive appearance of the mitral flow (E/A > 2) may be observed, due to the very rapid relaxation (hypernormal). In contrast, in older subjects (over 70 years of age),

---

Box 9.5   Pitfalls relating to the evaluation of the mitral flow using Doppler

Technical pitfalls
- Site selected for Doppler recording: at the mitral annulus or at the opening of the valves (frequent underestimation of the early diastolic velocities at the annular level)

- Poor alignment of the Doppler beam with the mitral flow (underestimation of the velocities)

- Imprecise measurement of the deceleration time of the E wave (time from the peak of the E wave to the intersection of the descending slope of the E wave with the baseline)

Diagnostic pitfalls
- Presence of factors that may modify the appearance of the mitral flow: age, load conditions, contractility, relaxation and compliance of the left ventricle, heart rate, mitral stenosis, mitral regurgitation, left bundle branch block, pacemaker

- Confusion between the pseudonormal mitral flow and the normal mitral flow

- Possibility of evolution from one mitral flow profile to another in the same patient

- Interpretation of the mitral flow appearance without taking the filling pressures into account

Table 9.3   Factors modifying the Doppler left ventricular filling parameters

Factor	E wave	A wave	E/A	DT	IVRT
Abnormal relaxation	↓	↑	↓	↑	↑
Impaired compliance	↑	↓	↑	↓	↓
Age	↓	↑	↓	↑	↑
Preload ↓ (hypovolaemia)	↓		↓	↑	↑
Preload ↑ (hypervolaemia)	↑		↑	↓	↓
Afterload ↑	↓		↓	↑	
Inspiration	↓	↓		↓	↑
Expiration	↑	↑		↑	↓
Tachycardia		↑	↓		
Bradycardia		↓	↑		
Left bundle branch block	↓	↑	↓		
Mitral regurgitation	↑		↑		

↑, increase; ↓, decrease; DT, deceleration time; IVRT, isovolumic relaxation time.

it is common to observe abnormal relaxation of the mitral flow (profile I) in a normal heart. In fact, this is a 'physiological' evolution of left ventricular filling with age. Therefore, a normal appearance of the mitral flow recorded in an older patient is most probably pathological (high probability of pseudonormalization).

With regard to the heart rate, the fusion of the E and A waves of the mitral flow in cases of sinus tachycardia (heart rate > 100 beats/min) should be noted. A carotid sinus massage, which can separate the E and A waves, is useful in this situation. Measurement of the mitral DT and the Em/Ea ratio is sometimes possible. Atrial fibrillation leads to the disappearance of the mitral A wave (see Fig. 9.4). The usual parameters (E/A, MAd) are therefore useless. The only parameters that can be analysed in this situation are the mitral DT, Em/Pv and Em/Ea (see page 187).

Among the conduction abnormalities, left bundle branch block leads to a reduction in the E/A ratio, and first-degree atrioventricular block results in a fusion of the E and A waves. Associated mitral regurgitation should always be taken into account in the interpretation of the mitral flow, as it may increase the A wave velocity and the E/A ratio. Finally, mitral flow profile II (pseudonormal appearance) may be difficult to distinguish from a normal profile (see page 181).

Isovolumic relaxation time
The isovolumic relaxation time (IVRT) of the LV is measured using pulsed or continuous wave Doppler and the apical four-chamber view, in one of two ways:

- from the aortic closing click to the mitral opening click (normal value 90 ± 20 ms) (Fig. 9.7)

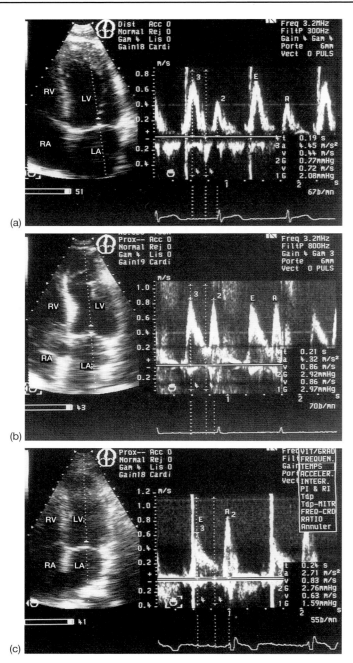

Figure 9.6 'Physiological' evolution of mitral flow with age: (a) young subject, E > A, deceleration time (DT) = 190 ms; (b) subject aged 60 years, E = A, DT = 210 ms; (c) subject aged 75 years, E < A, DT = 240 ms. LA, left atrium; LV, left ventricle; RA, right atrium; RV, right ventricle.

- from the aortic closing click to the beginning of the mitral flow that precedes the mitral click (normal value 70 ± 10 ms).

With pulsed Doppler, the sample volume is small (around 4 mm) and should be positioned between the outflow and LV inflow tracts. The pitfalls encountered when evaluating the IVRT are principally due to the factors that can modify its length, such as age, load conditions, left ventricular relaxation and compliance, and respiration (see Table 9.3). By completing the measurements of the mitral flow, IVRT plays a part in the differential diagnosis of the haemodynamic profiles of diastolic dysfunction of the LV (see Table 9.2).

Pulmonary venous flow
The pulmonary venous flow (PVF) can be analysed in 80–97% of patients using Doppler in the transthoracic approach. Normal PVF is biphasic, comprising (Figs 9.8 and 9.9):

- two positive waves, one systolic (S), due to the relaxation of the LA and the ventricular contraction, and the other diastolic (D), corresponding to the atrial emptying
- one negative end-diastolic wave (A) during atrial systole.

The parameters that can be used to analyse the diastolic function of the LV are:

- the S/D ratio (normal value > 1)
- the amplitude of the A wave (PA) (normal value < 35 cm/s)

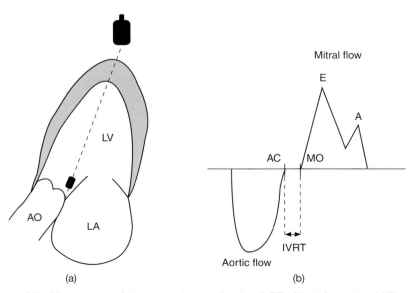

Figure 9.7   Measurement of the isovolumic relaxation time (IVRT) of the left ventricle. (a) The Doppler sample volume straddles the aorta and the mitral valve (apical cross-section of two left chambers with the aorta). (b) The IVRT is measured between the aortic closing (AC) click and the mitral opening (MO) click. AO, aorta; LA, left atrium; LV, left ventricle.

- the duration of the A wave (PAd); normally, the duration of the pulmonary A wave (venous emptying) is shorter than that of the A wave of the mitral flow (atrial emptying), PAd < MAd
- the deceleration time of the D wave (DDT) (normal > 220 ms).

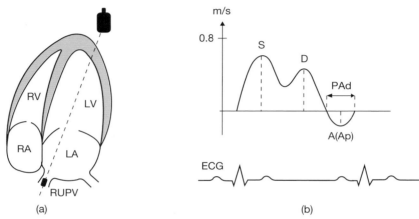

(a)   (b)

Figure 9.8   Echo Doppler examination of the normal pulmonary venous flow (PVF). (a) The Doppler sample volume is inside the right upper pulmonary vein (RUPV). (b) Schematic appearance of the PVF recorded using pulsed Doppler. Measurements: maximum S/D velocity ratio; amplitude (A(Ap)) and duration (PAd) of the A wave. LA, left atrium; LV, left ventricle; RA, right atrium; RV, right ventricle.

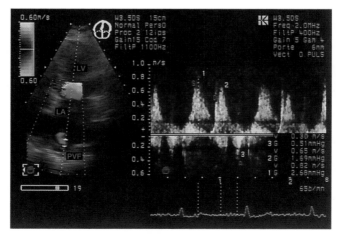

Figure 9.9   Normal pulmonary venous flow (PVF) recorded using transthoracic colour and pulsed Doppler (S wave 82 cm/s, D wave 65 cm/s, A wave 30 cm/s). LA, left atrium; LV, left ventricle.

Doppler study of the PVF assists in the differentiation of the diastolic dysfunction profiles of the LV (see Table 9.2 and Figs 9.10 and 9.11). Thanks to the combination of the parameters and to the analysis of the mitral flow and the pulmonary venous flow, it is possible to reliably obtain the left ventricular filling pressures (see page 181). When the diastolic pressure of the LV increases, the S wave decreases and the A wave increases in duration and amplitude, and may exceed the duration of the mitral A wave. The pitfalls relating to the evaluation of the PVF using Doppler are summarized in Box 9.6. The modification of the normal PVF velocities with age particularly concerns the D wave.

Propagation velocity of the mitral flow

The propagation velocity (Pv) of the mitral flow is measured using colour M-mode Doppler (Fig. 9.12). The normal value of Pv is > 45 cm/s in middle-aged adults and > 55 cm/s in younger subjects. The Pv value is a reflection of the left ventricular filling during early diastole (Fig. 9.13). In fact, the slope of the filling velocities of the LV in colour M-mode is linked to the ventricular relaxation. The pitfalls relating to recording and measuring the Pv of the mitral flow are summarized in Box 9.7. The Pv is an index of LV relaxation that is relatively inde-

---

Box 9.6   Pitfalls when evaluating the pulmonary venous flow (PVF) using Doppler

Failure to observe the PVF recording conditions
- Detection of the venous flow using 2D colour Doppler

- Doppler sample volume of 2–4 mm, positioned inside the pulmonary vein (1–2 cm before the opening into the left atrium)

- Doppler gains and filters adjusted to the minimum

- Spectral displacement velocity of 100 mm/s

- Measurements made at end of respiration

- Averaging of several cycles

Physiological PVF variations
- Age: ↓↓ D, ↑ S and A, but PA < 35 cm/s and PAd < MAd

- Heart rate: 'telescoping' of the S and D waves in cases of tachycardia

- Respiration: ↓ inspiratory minimum of the anteretrograde flows

Factors modifying the PVF
- Load conditions, relaxation and compliance of the left ventricle, volume of the left atrium

- Atrial fibrillation (disappearance of PA wave)

- Major mitral regurgitation (systolic reflux in the pulmonary veins leading to a negation of the S wave)

↑, increased; ↓, decreased; PA, amplitude of the A wave; PAd, duration of the A wave of pumonary venous flow; MAd, duration of the mitral A wave.

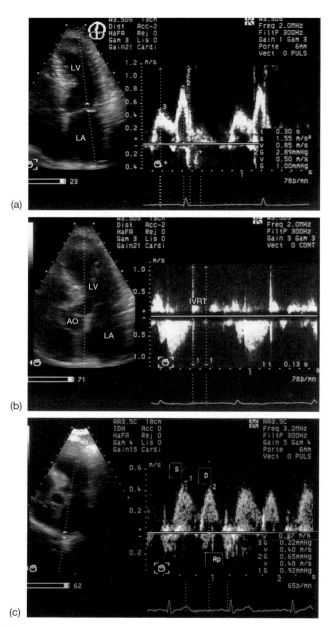

Figure 9.10 Profile I of diastolic left ventricular dysfunction (abnormal relaxation with elevated filling pressures). (a) Mitral fow: E/A = 0.59, deceleration time (DT) = 300 ms. (b) Isovolumic relaxation time (IVRT) = 130 ms. (c) Pulmonary venous flow: S/D = 1.2, amplitude of A wave (PA) = 37 cm/s, PAd > MAd. AO, aorta; LA, left atrium; LV, left ventricle; MAd, duration of mitral A wave; PAd, duration of A wave of pulmonary venous flow.

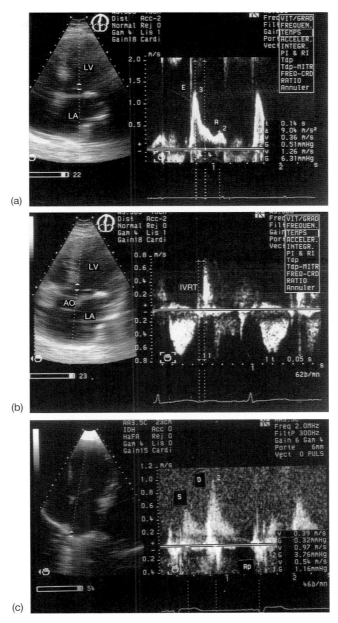

Figure 9.11 Profile III of diastolic left ventricular dysfunction (impaired compliance). (a) Mitral flow: E/A = 3.5, deceleration time (DT) = 140 ms. (b) Isovolumic relaxation time (IVRT) = 50 ms. (c) Pulmonary venous flow (PVF): S/D = 0.55, amplitude of A wave (PA) = 39 cm/s, PAd > MAd (C). AO, aorta; LA, left atrium; LV, left ventricle MAd, duration of mitral A wave; PAd, duration of the A wave of pulmonary venous flow.

pendent of the load conditions (preload in particular, Valsalva, glyceryl trinitrate) and heart rate. The patient's age has little influence on the value of Pv (moderate decrease in Pv with age). However, the value of Pv depends on the systolic function of the LV (positive correlation with the LV ejection fraction). Measurement of the Pv is useful in order to distinguish a normal mitral flow (where Pv

---

Box 9.7   Pitfalls when evaluating the propagation velocity (Pv) of the mitral flow using colour M-mode

Failure to observe Pv recording conditions
- Use of the apical four-chamber cross-section
- 2D colour sector positioned over the mitral flow up to the apex
- Zero line of the velocity scale displaced upwards (aliasing level 30–40 cm/s)
- Colour M-mode cursor applied to the 2D colour imaging in order to align it as closely as possible with the mitral flow
- Rapid displacement velocity using colour M-mode (100 mm/s)
- Cine mode and zoom usable

Imprecise measurement of the Pv
- On the aliasing slope of the early diastolic propagation of the mitral flow (blue–red interface)
- From the beginning of the mitral valve opening (detected on the mitral M-mode echo)
- At the minimum height of 4 cm

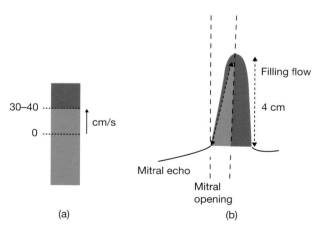

Figure 9.12   Colour M-mode Doppler examination of the propagation velocity (Pv) of the mitral flow. (a) Zero line of velocity scale displaced upwards (aliasing level 30–40 cm/s). (b) Recording of the left ventricular early diastolic filling flow in colour M-mode. Measurement of Pv from the beginning of mitral opening on the aliasing slope (blue–red interface) at the minimum height of 4 cm.

is normal) from a pseudonormal mitral flow (where Pv is lowered). The Em/Pv ratio is a simple tool for:

- identifying patients who have a pseudonormal profile (Box 9.8)
- evaluating the LV end-diastolic filling pressure (Box 9.9).

Doppler tissue imaging of the mitral annulus

Doppler tissue imaging (DTI), in pulsed mode, of the mitral annulus enables the displacement velocities of the mitral annulus to be analysed (Fig. 9.14).

The pitfalls relating to this analysis are associated with a lack of rigour in the examination methodology (Box 9.10) and the incorrect interpretation of the

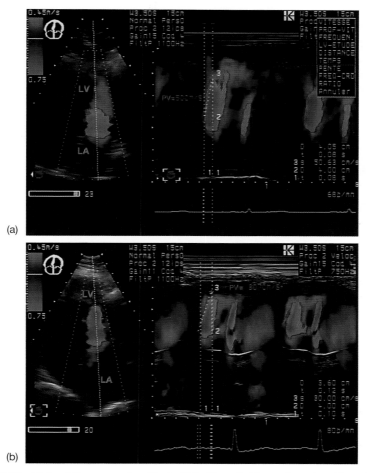

(a)

(b)

Figure 9.13   Study of the propagation velocity (Pv) of the mitral flow using colour M-mode: (a) normal appearance (Pv = 50 cm/s); (b) pathological appearance (Pv = 30 cm/s). LA, left atrium; LV, left ventricle.

Box 9.8   Doppler elements that suggest pseudonormal mitral flow

Mitral flow
- Exclusive reduction in the E wave during tests: Valsalva, glyceryl trinitrate (see Fig. 9.17)

Pulmonary venous flow
- Increase in the D wave: S/D < 1
- Increase in the pulmonary A wave: PA > 35 cm/s
- Increase in the duration of the pulmonary A wave: PAd > MAd

Mitral colour M-mode
- Reduction in the propagation velocity of the mitral flow: Pv < 45 cm/s
- Increase in Em/Pv > 10%

Mitral annular Doppler tissue imaging
- Reduction in the early diastolic displacement velocity of the mitral annulus: Ea < 8 cm/s
- Increase in Em/Ea > 10%

Box 9.9   Doppler values that support an elevation of left ventricular end-diastolic pressure

Mitral flow
- E/A > 2 (n > 1)
- EDT < 130 ms (n > 150 ms)

Pulmonary venous flow
- PAd – MAd > 20 ms (n < 0)
- DDT < 160 ms (n > 220 ms)

Mitral propagation velocity
- Em/Pv > 2.5 (n < 1.5)

Mitral annular velocity
- Em/Ea > 15 (n < 8)

---

data collected. The velocity curve recorded at the level of the mitral annulus in the pulsed DTI mode comprises three waves in the normal subject in sinus rhythm (Fig. 9.15):

- a positive systolic wave (Sa) corresponding to the displacement of the mitral annulus towards the apex of the heart (Sa = 9.7 ± 1.9 cm/s)
- two negative waves due to the displacement of the mitral annulus towards the base of the heart: early diastolic (Ea = 16 ± 3.7 cm/s) and end-diastolic (Aa = 10.9 ± 2 cm/s).

In practice, the normal appearance of the mitral annular velocities is an Ea wave > 8 cm/s (normal adult) or > 10 cm/s (normal youth) and an Ea/Aa ratio > 1 (normal 1.51 ± 0.47). The mitral annular velocities can be recorded at any level of the mitral annulus, but the velocities of the lateral part of the annulus appear to be less dependent on the load conditions than those of the septal part. The early diastolic displacement velocity of the mitral annulus (Ea) is not

---

Box 9.10   Pitfalls when analysing the mitral annulus using Doppler spectral tissue imaging (DTI)

Failure to observe mitral annular DTI methodology
- From the apical four-chamber view
- Volume measurement placed at the level of the mitral annulus (lateral or septal)
- Doppler sample volume of 8–10 mm
- Filters and gains adjusted to the minimum
- Reduced velocity scale: ≈ 20 cm/s
- Displacement velocity of the correctly adjusted spectrum

Factors modifying the mitral annular velocities
- Age of patient examined
- Left ventricular preload
- Myocardial ischaemia or necrosis
- Wall hypertrophy

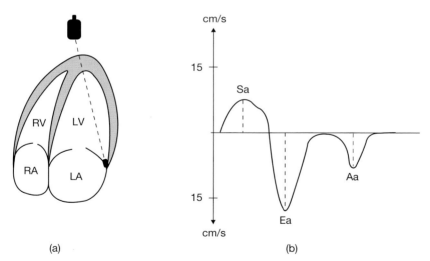

(a)   (b)

Figure 9.14   Doppler tissue imaging (DTI) applied to the mitral annulus. (a) Position of the Doppler sample volume at the level of the lateral mitral annulus (apical four-chamber view). (b) Schematic drawing of the mitral annular velocity curve recorded using pulsed DTI. Measurements: maximum velocities of the Sa, Ea and Aa waves. LA, left atrium; LV, left ventricle; RA, right atrium; RV, right ventricle.

greatly influenced by the patient's age (moderate decrease in Ea with age) or by the load conditions (particularly the preload). On the other hand, it is influenced by myocardial ischaemia or necrosis affecting the annular zone, and by wall hypertrophy of the LV (decreased Ea).

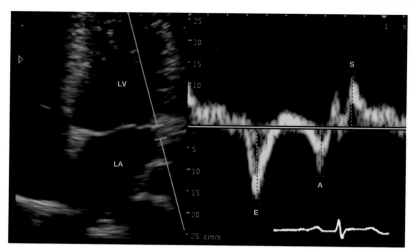

Figure 9.15 Doppler tissue imaging in pulsed mode applied to the lateral mitral annulus (Imagic system, Kontron-Esaote). Spectral curve of the normal mitral annular velocities (Ea = 17 cm/s, Aa = 11 cm/s; Sa = 12 cm/s, Ea/Aa = 1.5). LA, left atrium; LV, left ventricle.

When applied to the mitral annulus DTI is an extremely valuable tool for evaluating the LV diastolic function (Fig. 9.16). The clinical advantages of this technique are:

- the early detection of abnormal relaxation of the LV (inversion of the Ea/Aa ratio)
- the differentiation between a normal and a pseudonormal mitral flow profile (see Box 9.8)
- the evaluation of the LV filling pressures (see Box 9.9).

Differential diagnosis between pseudonormal and normal mitral flow

Pseudonormal mitral flow is characteristic of haemodynamic profile II (see Table 9.2). It is due to the slowing of the relaxation of the LV and an elevation of the ventricular filling pressures, masking a relaxation abnormality. The classic Doppler examination shows a 'pseudonormalization' of the mitral flow, with normal E/A, DT and IVRT. This pseudonormal appearance is associated with many pitfalls in diagnosis, as it is falsely reassuring. There are two ways in which pseudonormal mitral flow can be identified:

- by unmasking abnormal relaxation through the Valsalva manoeuvre or the glyceryl trinitrate test, and by measuring parameters such as Pv and Ea (Figs 9.17 and 9.18)
- by demonstrating an elevation of the filling pressures through an analysis of the pulmonary venous flow and combined measurements (Em/Pv and Em/Ea).

The Doppler measurements that argue in favour of pseudonormal mitral flow are summarized in Box 9.9.

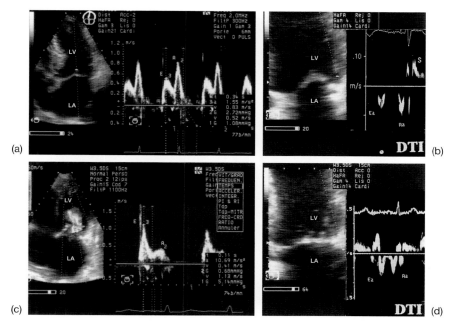

Figure 9.16 Diastolic left ventricular dysfunction viewed using (a, c) conventional pulsed Doppler (mitral flow) and (b, d) Doppler tissue imaging (mitral annular DTI). (a, b) Profile I (abnormal relaxation): (a) E/A = 0.6, deceleration time (DT) = 340 ms; (b) Ea = 6 cm/s, Ea/Aa = 0.54. (c, d) Profile III (impaired compliance): (c) E/A = 2.7, DT = 100 ms; (d) Ea = 3 cm/s, Ea/Aa = 1.2. LA, left atrium; LV, left ventricle.

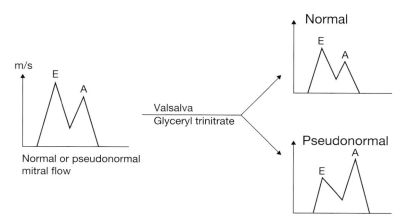

Figure 9.17 Differentiation of the normal from the pseudonormal mitral flow (MF) during the Valsalva manoeuvre or testing with glyceryl trinitrate. Note: there are equivalent reductions in the E and A waves when the mitral flow is normal; there is a reduction in the E wave only when the mitral flow is pseudonormal.

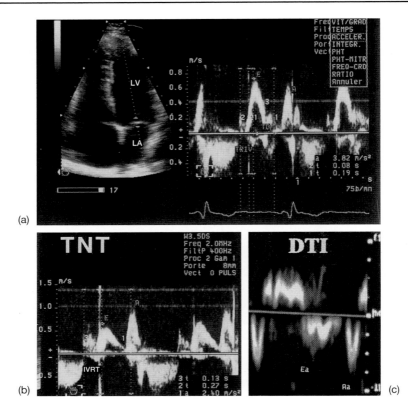

Figure 9.18 Detection of left ventricular diastolic dysfunction in (a) the presence of a pseudo-normal mitral flow. Abnormal left ventricular relaxation disturbance illustrated using (b) the glyceryl trinitrate test (inversion of the E/A ratio of the mitral flow) and (b) mitral annular DTI (inversion of the Ea/Aa ratio). LA, left atrium; LV, left ventricle; IVRT, isovolumic relaxation time.

Estimation of the left ventricular filling pressures

The LV filling pressures reflect the state of the atrioventricular diastolic filling. It is possible to estimate the pressures using the following echo Doppler parameters:

- mitral flow: E/A ratio, E wave deceleration time (EDT)
- pulmonary venous flow: A wave duration (PAd) compared with the mitral A wave duration (MAd) (difference: PAd – MAd), pulmonary D wave deceleration time (DDT)
- mitral flow propagation velocities in colour M-mode Doppler (Pv): E mitral/Pv ratio (Em/Pv)
- early diastolic displacement velocity of the mitral annulus in DTI (Ea): E mitral/E annular ratio (Em/Ea).

The Doppler measurements that suggest an elevation of LV filling pressures are summarized in Box 9.9.

The use of the combined parameters (Em/Pv, Em/Ea) for estimating the left ventricular end-diastolic pressure is particularly advantageous in the case of atrial fibrillation, as the other parameters may be erroneous in this situation. However, the normal values of the ratios (Em/Pv, Em/Ea) cover a rather broad range.

The pitfalls associated with using echo Doppler to estimate the LV filling pressures are due to:

- the examination methodology – recording and measuring different diastolic echo Doppler parameters
- the interpretation of the results obtained.

In fact, there are several factors that modify the LV filling pressures, such as:

- the elastic properties of the myocardium
- the LV geometry (hypertrophy, dilatation)
- the quality of the ventricular relaxation
- pericardial constraint
- coronary filling.

These factors should be taken into consideration when interpreting the results of the echo Doppler examination of an individual. The actual evaluation of the LV filling pressures therefore remains complex, and is particularly difficult in the average patient (Em/Pv between 1.5 and 2.5, Em/Ea between 8 and 15). For the considerable number of patients who fall into this group, it is important to make use of as many filling parameters as possible, in particular the variation in E/A after Valsalva, the value of the difference PAd – MAd, etc., without forgetting other parameters such as the systolic pulmonary pressure or the cardiac output. A synthesis of this information, repetition of the examinations and the clinical data make it possible to define better a patient's haemodynamic state.

PITFALLS WHEN EVALUATING THE SYSTOLIC AND DIASTOLIC FUNCTION OF THE RIGHT VENTRICLE

Evaluation of right ventricular function using Doppler echocardiography is made more difficult by:

- the often poor definition of the endocardium of the right ventricle (RV) when determining the ventricular contours (poor lateral resolution, highly trabeculated apex, subject with low echogenicity)
- the complex geometry of the RV, which is difficult to model (crescent-shaped appearance wrapped around the LV, or bellows-shaped)
- respiratory variations in the size of the RV (increased during inspiration)
- a physiological asynchrony of the right ventricular free wall contraction
- interference of the LV on the RV by means of the interventricular septum, the pericardium and the pulmonary circulation
- the presence of other factors influencing the right ventricular function (patient's age, heart rate, load conditions, therapy, etc.).

Several echo Doppler parameters are used in the analysis of the systolic and diastolic function of the right ventricle (Box 9.11). The parameters are influ-

Box 9.11   Normal echo Doppler parameters for analysing the systolic and diastolic functions of the right ventricle

Systolic parameters
- Ejection fraction
- Surface shortening fraction
- Pulmonary pre-ejection time
- Systolic excursion of the tricuspid annulus
- Maximum velocity of the tricuspid annular systolic wave
- Duration of the right ventricular isovolumic contraction

Diastolic parameters
- Tricuspid flow profile
- Hepatic venous flow profile
- Tricuspid annular diastolic displacement velocity
- Right ventricular isovolumic relaxation time

enced by the many factors mentioned above, and familiarity with these factors is necessary in order to avoid incorrect interpretation of the results.

Analysis of right ventricular systolic function
Analysis of the systolic function of the RV is based on echocardiographic data (2D) and Doppler data (spectral and tissue imaging).

Ejection fraction
The ejection fraction (EF) reflects the right ventricular pumping function in the absence of significant tricuspid regurgitation. The EF of the RV is calculated using the end-diastolic volume (EDV, a reflection of the preload) and the end-systolic volume (ESV, a reflection of the afterload) of the RV according to the formula:

$$EF = \frac{EDV - ESV}{EDV} \times 100 \text{ (normal > 48\%)}$$

This method requires measurements to be made in several 2D cross-sectional planes, according to the volumetric model applied to the planimetric measurement of the end-diastolic and end-systolic surface areas of the RV. The advantages of this method in clinical practice are few, due to the difficulty of its execution.

Surface shortening fraction
The surface shortening fraction (SSF) of the RV is a dimension equivalent to the ejection fraction. It is calculated using the end-diastolic (EDS) and end-systolic (ESS) surface areas of the RV measured planimetrically in the apical four-chamber view (Fig. 9.19):

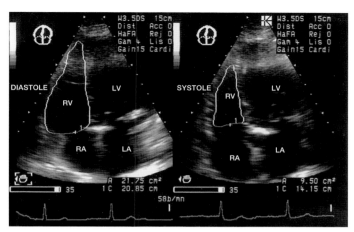

Figure 9.19 Evaluation of the surface shortening fraction (SSF) of the right ventricle (RV) using the planimetric method in the apical four-chamber view during diastole and systole (end-diastolic surface area (EDS) = 21.7 cm², end-systolic surface area (ESS) = 9.5 cm², SSF = 57%). LA, left atrium; LV, left ventricle; RA, right atrium.

$$SSF = \frac{EDS - ESS}{EDS} \times 100 \ (normal > 50\%)$$

This is a simple parameter to measure but, like the EF of the RV, it is also dependent on the ventricular load conditions.

Pulmonary pre-ejection time

The pulmonary pre-ejection time is measured from the beginning of the QRS of the ECG until the beginning of the pulmonary flow recorded using pulsed Doppler (normal value: 70–90 ms). It is lengthened in cases of right ventricular systolic dysfunction (Fig. 9.20).

Parameters measured using Doppler tissue imaging

The parameters measured using DTI principally involve:

- the amplitude of the systolic displacement wave of the tricuspid annular plane, studied using M-mode (normal maximum systolic excursion 20 mm)
- the maximum velocity of the systolic displacement wave of the tricuspid annular plane, studied using pulsed Doppler (normal maximum systolic wave 14 cm/s).

Systolic dysfunction of the RV leads to a reduction in the detailed values of these parameters in DTI.

Analysis of right ventricular diastolic function

The analysis of right ventricular filling is based on the study of:

- the tricuspid flow and the hepatic venous flow, using classic pulsed Doppler

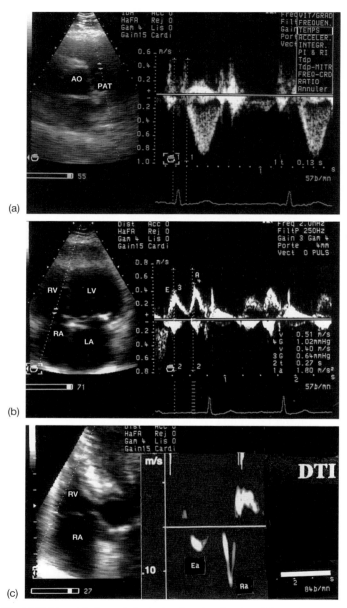

Figure 9.20   (a) Right ventricular systolic dysfunction: lengthening of the pulmonary pre-ejection time (130 ms) over the pulmonary flow, recorded using pulsed Doppler. (b) Right ventricular diastolic dysfunction: inversion of the E/A ratio (0.78) with a lengthened deceleration time (270 ms) of the tricuspid flow, recorded using pulsed Doppler, and (c) with inversion of the Ea/Aa ratio (0.6) of the tricuspid annular velocities recorded using DTI. AO, aorta; LA, left atrium; LV, left ventricle; PAT, pulmonary arterial trunk; RA, right atrium; RV, right ventricle.

- the diastolic displacement velocities of the tricuspid annulus, using DTI
- the isovolumic relaxation time of the RV, obtained from the difference between the time separating the R wave of the ECG from the tricuspid opening, and the time separating the R wave from the end of pulmonary arterial ejection.

Tricuspid flow

The velocity curve of the normal tricuspid flow is comparable to that of the mitral flow. It is biphasic, being composed of the E wave, which corresponds to rapid filling of the RV, and the A wave, which is due to the contraction of the right atrium. Normally, the E wave is broader than the A wave. The E and A waves increase during inspiration and decrease during expiration (Fig. 9.21).

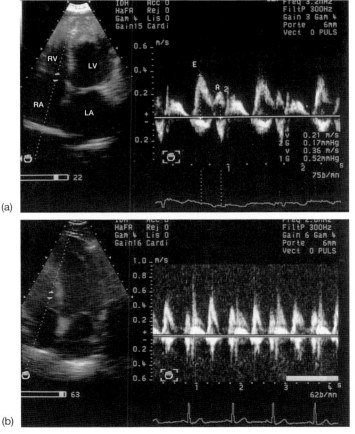

Figure 9.21   (a) Normal tricuspid flow (E/A > 1) recorded using pulsed Doppler.
(b) Physiological respiratory variations of the tricuspid flow. LA, left atrium; LV, left ventricle; RA, right atrium; RV, right ventricle.

These waves must therefore be measured either during apnoea or by taking the average of five consecutive tricuspid flows measured during normal respiration.

Hepatic venous flow

The hepatic venous flow curve is similar to the curve of the pressure in the right atrium. The curve is quadriphasic, being composed of:

- two negative waves (anteretrograde flows), one systolic (S) and one diastolic (D)
- two positive waves (retrograde flows), one ventricular (V) and one atrial (A).

Normally, the velocity of the S wave is greater than that of the D wave (Figs 9.22 and 9.23).

The hepatic venous flow varies with respiration: during inspiration the velocity of the S and D waves increases, and that of the V and A waves decreases; at the beginning of expiration, the situation is reversed.

Diastolic displacement velocities of the tricuspid annulus

Normally, the velocity curve recorded at the level of the tricuspid annulus using DTI comprises three waves: one systolic wave (S), and two diastolic waves (Ea and Aa). Normally, the ratio of the annular velocities Ea/Aa is > 1 (Fig. 9.24).

Analysis of the right ventricular diastolic parameters allows two types of abnormal right ventricular diastolic function to be identified: abnormal right ventricular relaxation and impaired compliance (Table 9.4 and see Fig. 9.20).

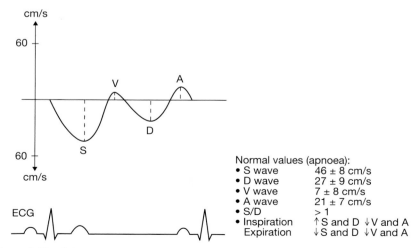

Normal values (apnoea):
- S wave   46 ± 8 cm/s
- D wave   27 ± 9 cm/s
- V wave   7 ± 8 cm/s
- A wave   21 ± 7 cm/s
- S/D   > 1
- Inspiration   ↑S and D ↓V and A
- Expiration   ↓S and D ↓V and A

Figure 9.22 Schematic drawing of the normal hepatic venous flow. Measurement of the maximum velocities of the S, D, V and A waves.

Summary

In conclusion, the complexity of the systolic and diastolic function of the RV requires careful analysis of the echo Doppler parameters used. Results from the different methods for evaluating right ventricular function should be compared with one another in order to increase the reliability of the examination outcome and the coherence of the echocardiographic results both within themselves and with the rest of the clinical presentation.

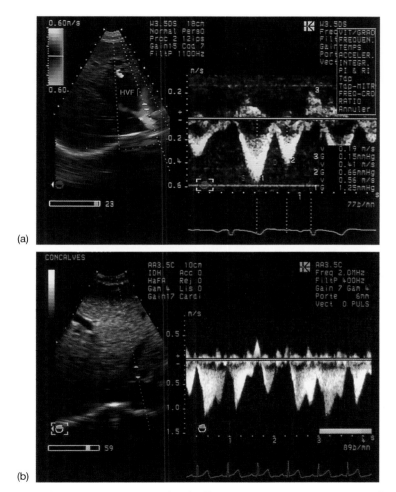

(a)

(b)

Figure 9.23   (a) Normal hepatic venous flow (HVF) recorded using transthoracic pulsed Doppler in the subcostal cross-section (S = 56 cm/s, D = 41 cm/s, A = 19 cm/s). (b) Physiological respiratory variations in the HVF.

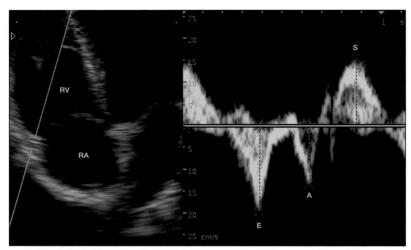

Figure 9.24 Doppler tissue imaging in pulsed mode applied to the lateral tricuspid annulus (Imagic system, Kontron-Esaote). Spectral curve of the normal tricuspid annular velocities (Ea = 20 cm/s, Aa = 13 cm/s, Sa = 15 cm/s). RA, right atrium; RV, right ventricle.

Table 9.4   Characteristics of the two types of right ventricular diastolic dysfunction: abnormal relaxation and impaired compliance

Parameter	Abnormal relaxation	Impaired compliance
Tricuspid flow	E/A < 1 DT > 250 ms	E/A > 1.5 DT < 200 ms
Hepatic venous flow	S ↑ (> 40 cm/s) D ↓ (< 25 cm/s) or annulled (S/D >> 1)	A ↑ (> 25 cm/s) then S ↓ (< 30 cm/s) or annulled and D ↑ (> 35 m/s) (S/D < 1)
Right ventricular isovolumic relaxation time	> 80 ms	< 60 ms
Early diastolic tricuspid annular velocity	Ea ↓ (Ea/Aa < 1)	Ea ↓↓ (Ea/Aa < 1)

↑ ,increased; ↓, decreased.

10
Pulmonary arterial pressures

Echocardiography coupled with Doppler constitutes a validated, non-invasive and easily accessible method for evaluating the pulmonary arterial pressures (PAPs). The pitfalls of using echo Doppler in this scenario relate to:

- the detection and quantification of pulmonary arterial hypertension (PAHT)
- the differential diagnosis between pre- and postcapillary PAHT
- the interpretation of the PAP values.

DETECTION AND QUANTIFICATION OF PULMONARY ARTERIAL HYPERTENSION

The echocardiographic diagnosis of PAHT is based on the echocardiographic imaging data and the Doppler signs.

Echocardiographic signs

The presence of PAHT may entail a certain number of morphological modifications of the right chambers, which can be identified using echocardiography (Fig. 10.1):

- dilatation of the right ventricle and the pulmonary trunk
- hypertrophy of the right ventricular free wall
- more or less paradoxical movement of the interventricular septum
- dilatation of the inferior vena cava and the subhepatic veins
- M-mode anomaly of the pulmonary valve (absence of the 'a' wave; mid-systolic pulmonary closing).

The echocardiographic signs listed above are highly suggestive when PAHT is frank, but a normal or subnormal morphology of the right chambers does not in any way eliminate a diagnosis of PAHT. Moreover, the signs of PAHT are diversely associated, and all present numerous limitations and diagnostic pitfalls, namely:

- These signs are also seen with causes of right overload (e.g. interatrial communication, autonomous tricuspid valvulopathy).
- The importance of these signs depends not only on the severity of the PAHT, but also on its age, its permanent or paroxystic nature, and on the volume of a potential associated tricuspid regurgitation. In fact, this presentation is only characteristic in the presence of a marked PAHT (systolic PAP > 50 mmHg). The repercussion on the right chambers is slight, or even absent in certain cases of PAHT (e.g. in markedly depleted patients).

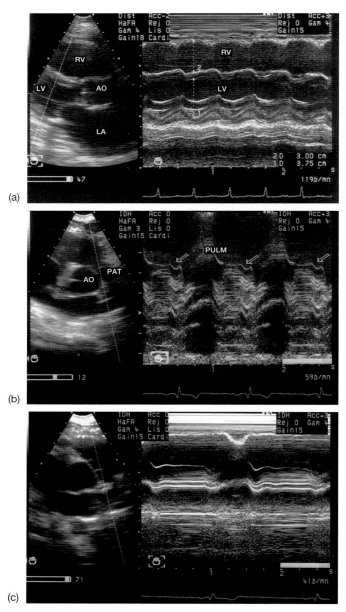

Figure 10.1 Echocardiographic signs of pulmonary arterial hypertension (PAHT). (a) Dilatation of the right ventricle (RV) (diastolic diameter = 30 mm; RV/LV ratio = 0.8) with a paradoxical septum. (b). Normal pulmonary 'a' wave recorded using M-mode. (c) Disappearance of the 'a' wave from the M-mode echocardiogram of the pulmonary valve. AO, aorta; LA, left atrium; LV, left ventricle; PAT, pulmonary arterial trunk;; PULM, pulmonic valve.

- The deformation of the interventricular septum may be variable: it may have a flat, or even inverted (known as 'paradoxical', a convex septal curvature towards the left ventricle) appearance in pressure overloads (PAHT); it has a straight appearance (flat in both systole and diastole) in volaemic overloads (major tricuspid regurgitation).
- Modifications of the pulmonary valve movement seen using M-mode, which indicate PAHT, have low specificity and low sensitivity.

In sinus rhythm, the reduction in, or even the absence of, the pulmonary 'a' wave may indicate an increase in the diastolic PAP. In the case of right ventricular failure associated with PAHT, the 'a' wave may reappear, due to the increase in the right ventricular filling pressures. Finally, continuous arrhythmia due to atrial fibrillation leads to a disappearance of the pulmonary 'a' wave. The partial mid-systolic closure of the pulmonary sigmoid valves observed in PAHT is equivalent to the mid-systolic notch of the pulmonary ejection flow recorded using pulsed Doppler (see page 203). In reality, the pulmonary M-mode signs are only present in frank PAHT (systolic PAP > 50 mmHg and/or average PAP > 20 mmHg).

In conclusion, all these echocardiographic criteria for evaluating the PAPs remain semiquantitative and are in fact surpassed by the Doppler criteria.

Doppler signs

The secure diagnosis of PAHT rests on the Doppler data, which make it possible to measure the PAPs precisely.

In practice, four methods are used to evaluate the PAPs with Doppler. These four methods are based on the analysis of the following flows:

- tricuspid regurgitation (TR)
- pulmonary regurgitation (PR)
- pulmonary ejection
- left-to-right shunt (interventricular and arterial canal communication).

The study of the TR and PR flows are unquestionably the two most commonly used methods.

Study of the tricuspid regurgitant flow

The flow due to TR may be used in the majority of patients due to the high frequency of TR noted in the presence of PAHT (80–90% of cases).

On the basis of the TR flow recorded using continuous Doppler, it is possible to evaluate the systolic PAP, using the maximum TR velocity (Box 10.1 and Fig. 10.2).

The advantage of the TR method is its reliability, as demonstrated by the excellent correlation between the values of the systolic PAP estimated using Doppler and the catheter method. Nevertheless, the TR method does involve errors and has limitations. The pitfalls that arise when using echo Doppler in this situation are technical and/or diagnostic in nature (Box 10.2).

> **Box 10.1   Formulae for calculating the systolic (PAP$_s$), diastolic (PAP$_d$) and mean (PAP$_m$) pulmonary arterial pressures using the different flows**
>
> **Tricuspid regurgitant flow (TR)**
> PAP$_s$ = 4V TR^2 + RAP
>
> **Pulmonary regurgitant flow (PR)**
> PAP$_d$ = 4V_{ed} PR^2 + RAP
>
> PAP$_m$ = 4V_{pd} PR^2 + RAP
>
> PAP$_s$ = 3PAP$_m$ − 2PAP$_d$
>
> **Tricuspid and pulmonary regurgitant flow**
> PAP$_m$ = ⅓ PAP$_s$ + ⅔ PAP$_d$
>
> **Pulmonary ejection flow**
> PAP$_m$ > 20 mmHg if acceleration time < 100 ms
>
> **Interventricular communication flow (IVC)**
> PAP$_s$ = SAP − 4V IVC^2
>
> **Arterial canal (AC) flow**
> PAP$_s$ = SAP − 4V AC^2
>
> RAP, right atrial pressure; SAP, systolic arterial pressure; V, maximum velocity; V_{ed}, end-diastolic velocity; V_{pd}, early diastolic velocity.

Technical pitfalls

Confusion between a TR flow and a mitral regurgitation flow may occur when using continuous Doppler blind. In this situation, it is necessary to carry out a careful sweep from the mitral flow to the tricuspid flow via the aortic flow. In practice, continuous Doppler guided by 2D colour Doppler is used, making it possible to detect the TR visually.

Another technical pitfall arises from poor alignment of the ultrasound beam with the TR jet, leading to an underestimation of the maximum TR velocity, and therefore of the systolic PAP (Fig. 10.3). The ideal solution is to detect the origin of the TR jet by the high velocities in 2D colour Doppler, and then to align the Doppler line of sight over this jet. However, it is still recommended that continuous Doppler be used blind, in order to use as many projections as possible (apical, low parasternal, subcostal) and thus to obtain the highest possible values of the TR velocity. Errors in the measurement of the TR may also arise from a weak Doppler signal due to:

- a low-volume or highly eccentric TR jet, which is difficult to capture
- incorrect adjustment of the ultrasound machine (gains and filters in particular)
- limited echogenicity of the patient examined.

Another cause of errors is linked to a lack of averaging of the maximum TR velocities, in cases where atrial fibrillation causes these velocities to vary, or in

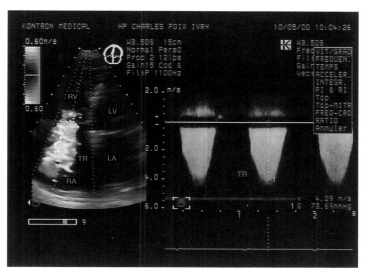

Figure 10.2 Measurement of pulmonary arterial pressures (PAPs) on the basis of the tricuspid regurgitation (TR) flow recorded in colour and continuous Doppler. V_{max} of TR = 4.3 m/s; D P syst RV/RA = 74 mmHg. Systolic PAP: 74 + 10 = 84 mmHg (severe pulmonary arterial hypertension) (estimating right arterial pressure at 10 mmHg). LA, left atrium; LV, left ventricle; RA, right atrium; RV, right ventricle.

Box 10.2   Pitfalls in the evaluation of the pulmonary pressures when using echo Doppler on the basis of the tricuspid regurgitation (TR) flow

Technical pitfalls
- Confusion between mitral regurgitation and TR

- Faulty alignment with the TR jet

- Weak Doppler signal

- Lack of averaging of TR velocities

Diagnostic pitfalls
- Errors in estimation of right arterial pressure

- Laminar TR

- Trivial TR

- Associated pulmonary stenosis

---

cases of major respiratory variations in the TR velocity. These respiratory variations are partly due to the variations in the pulmonary pressures, and partly to the changes in the angle between the ultrasound beam and the TR jet during respiratory movements. In these situations, the TR values should be averaged over 5 to 10 consecutive cardiac cycles.

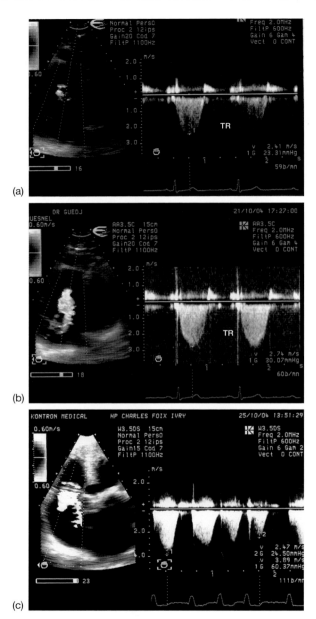

Figure 10.3 Causes of error in estimating the systolic pulmonary arterial pressures (PAPs) on the basis of the tricuspid regurgitation (TR) flow. (a) Poor alignment of the continuous Doppler beam with the TR jet, underestimating the maximum velocity of the TR jet (V_{max} = 2.4 m/s) and therefore the systolic PAP (PAP$_s$ = 23 + RAP). (b) With correct alignment: V_{max} = 2.74 m/s, PAP$_s$ = 30 + RAP. (c) Variation in the TR V_{max} (and therefore in PAP$_s$) in the presence of an atrial fibrillation. RAP, right atrial pressure.

Diagnostic pitfalls

Mistaken estimation of the right atrial pressure

Classically, the systolic PAP is evaluated by adding an arbitrary value of the systolic right atrial pressure (RAP) to the right atrioventricular pressure during systole, in the absence of pulmonary stenosis.

An error in the estimation of the RAP constitutes an essential diagnostic pitfall. In fact, there is no robust method for the non-invasive measurement of the pressure in the right atrium. In order to evaluate this pressure, different approaches have been proposed: the use of a fixed empirical value of 5 mmHg (in children) or 10 mmHg (in adults); or a modulated value according to the clinical or echocardiographic presentation. In fact, the RAP is estimated as a function of:

- the importance of the signs of right cardiac failure (slight 10 mmHg, moderate 15 mmHg, severe 20 mmHg)
- the degree of jugular vein distension (flat 5 mmHg, distended 10–15 mmHg, turgescent 15–20 mmHg)
- the diameter of the inferior vena cava and its respiratory variations
- the subhepatic venous flow
- the appearance of the tricuspid annular velocities in Doppler tissue imaging.

In practice, it is accepted that an arbitrary value of 10 mmHg be applied in the majority of adult subjects. However, in certain cases, the actual value of the RAP may be underestimated, requiring the addition of 15–25 mmHg to this value.

The choice of the value of the RAP may be guided by analysing the diameter of the inferior vena cava and its respiratory variations in the 2D mode (Table 10.1). This diameter should be measured in the 2 cm preceding the point where the inferior vena cava joins the right atrium, and during expiration (maximum value). Normally, the diameter is of the order of 18 ± 5 mm. The variations with respiration of the diameter of the inferior vena cava are quantified by calculating the shortening fraction of the diameter (caval index) according to the formula:

$$\text{Caval index} = \frac{\text{Expiratory diameter} - \text{Inspiratory diameter}}{\text{Expiratory diameter}}$$

When using this calculation, the smallest inspiratory diameter and the largest expiratory diameter are recorded, thus avoiding any Valsalva manoeuvre

Table 10.1 Evaluation of the right atrial pressure (RAP) on the basis of the inferior vena cava diameter and its variations with respiration (inspiratory caval index)

Diameter (mm)	Caval index (%)	RAP (mmHg)
< 15	≈ 100	0–5
12–25	> 50	5–10
> 25	< 50	10–20
> 25	≈ 0	> 20

(Fig. 10.4). The normal value of the caval index is in the range 50–100%. In practice, an index below 50% suggests an elevation of the RAP (> 10 mmHg).

The echocardiographic analysis of the inferior vena cava can be limited for technical reasons (accessibility of the vein only by means of the subcostal approach), in cases of assisted ventilation (caval index not usable) and in high-level athletes (in whom the diameter of the inferior vena cave may exceed 25 mm).

The RAP may also be evaluated on the basis of the subhepatic venous flow (SHVF). The SHVF velocity curve recorded using pulsed Doppler in the subcostal approach is comparable to that of the pressure in the right atrium (see Fig. 9.22). This velocity curve can be used to calculate the systolic fraction (SF)

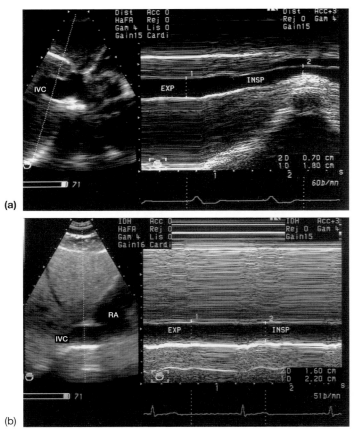

(a)

(b)

Figure 10.4   Study of the inferior vena cava (IVC) using 2D M-mode echocardiography. (a) Normal IVC: expiratory diameter = 18 mm, caval index = 61%. (b) Dilated IVC (pulmonary arterial hypertension): expiratory diameter = 22 mm, caval index = 27%). EXP, expiration; INSP, inspiration; RA, right atrium.

of the SHVF using the VTIs of the systolic (VTI_s) and diastolic (VTI_d) waves of the flow:

$$SF = \frac{VTI_s}{VTI_s + VTI_d}$$

The RAP may then be calculated using the formula:

$$RAP = 21.6 - 24 \times FS$$

The use of this method for evaluating the RAP is limited, particularly in cases of atrial fibrillation or a massive TR.

The RAP may also be estimated by analysing the displacement velocities of the lateral tricuspid annulus using pulsed Doppler tissue imaging. An E/Ea ratio of > 6 predicts a RAP of ≥ 10 mmHg.

Finally, some authors have proposed calculating the systolic PAP on the basis of the sole velocity peak of the TR (V) recorded using continuous Doppler, according to the formula:

$$PAP_s = 1.23 \times 4V^2$$

Laminar tricuspid regurgitation
It is necessary to be familiar with the pitfall of laminar TR. This corresponds to a TR of large volume (massive TR) in 2D colour Doppler and associated with low TR velocities in continuous Doppler (< 2.5 m/s).

The analysis in pulsed Doppler at the level of the tricuspid orifice shows a laminar regurgitant flow, confirming the massive TR (Fig. 10.5). This massive laminar TR is due to the dilatation of the right chambers and the tricuspid annulus, secondary to a major PAHT, which renders the tricuspid valve incompetent (systolic hiatus). Therefore, in the case of this severe leak, there is a ventricularization of the atrial pressures, and the pressure of the right atrium, during both systole and diastole, is significantly increased.

This situation explains the underestimated values of the systolic PAP derived from the maximum velocity of the TR, as Bernoulli's simplified equation is no longer suitable (the velocity upstream of the regurgitant orifice can no longer be discounted). This error in the calculation of the systolic PAP on the basis of the maximum TR velocity is systematic if the leak is laminar. The classic calculation of the systolic PAP therefore ceases to be reliable (there is a risk of greatly underestimating the severity of PAHT) and should lead to the method being rejected. In this situation, analysis of the PR flow is preferable.

Trivial tricuspid regurgitation
This peculiarity of TR is rare but may represent a pitfall. It portrays a TR of high velocity but very low volume, giving a poorly defined, and therefore largely incomplete or poorly formed, spectral envelope. This trivial TR, which may be accompanied by major PAHT, is often difficult to explore using continuous Doppler coupled with imaging. It requires the use of a Pedoff probe and/or intra-cardiac contrast, which makes it possible to strengthen the image of the TR jet.

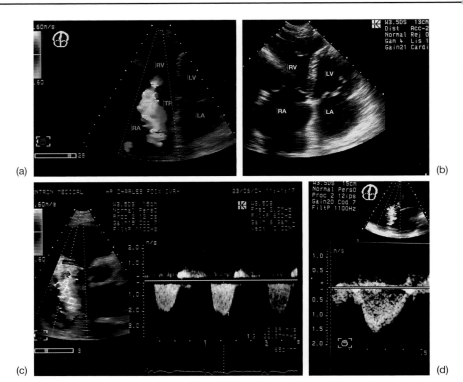

Figure 10.5   Laminar tricuspid regurgitation (TR). (a) Massive TR in colour Doppler. (b) Dilated right chambers, and systolic hiatus of the tricuspid valve in 2D. (c) Low velocity TR in continuous Doppler (2.4 m/s). (d) Laminar appearance (organized and enveloped) of the TR flow in pulsed Doppler. LA, left atrium; LV, left ventricle; RA, right atrium; RV, right ventricle.

Unknown associated pulmonary stenosis

Unknown associated pulmonary stenosis constitutes a significant cause of errors in the estimation of the systolic PAP on the basis of TR.

Classically, the maximum velocity of the TR can be used to obtain, by means of Bernoulli's simplified equation, the pressure gradient between the right atrium and the right ventricle. The systolic pressure of the right ventricle is calculated by adding the RAP to this gradient. This right ventricular pressure may be assimilated into the systolic PAP if there is no pulmonary stenosis. In fact, any modification to the systolic right ventricular pressure leads to a variation in the TR velocity.

In cases of associated pulmonary stenosis, the corresponding stenotic gradient should be subtracted from the systolic pressure of the right ventricle in order to obtain the actual systolic PAP. The absence of pulmonary stenosis should, therefore, be confirmed during the study of the PAHT.

Study of the pulmonary regurgitant flow

A study of the flow of PR makes it possible to calculate the pulmonary pressures in the absence of a measurable TR. The PR flow may be recorded using continuous Doppler in 60–75% of patients presenting with PAHT. The PR flow velocity reflects the diastolic pressure gradient between the pulmonary artery and the right ventricle, and its value is increased in PAHT. The early diastolic velocity (V_{pd}) and end-diastolic velocity (V_{ed}) are correlated with the mean (PAP_m) and diastolic (PAP_d) PAP values, respectively (Fig. 10.6(b)). In practice, an end-diastolic PR flow velocity above 1.5 m/s indicates PAHT. The systolic PAP (PAP_s) may be evaluated using the PR flow and an empirical formula (see Box 10.1). The pitfalls (technical and diagnostic) when using Doppler to evaluate the pulmonary pressures according to the PR method are summarized in Box 10.3.

Technical pitfalls

The technical pitfalls encountered when studying the PR flow are principally problems of PRs of low volume, or PRs not detectable in echo Doppler for various reasons (patient hypoechogenicity, imperfect visualization of the pulmon-

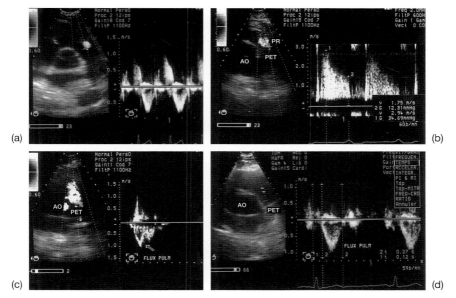

Figure 10.6 Study of the pulmonary flow in pulmonary arterial hypertension. (a) Physiological pulmonary regurgitation (PR) recorded using continuous Doppler. (b) PR with an early diastolic velocity of 2.9 m/s (gradient 33 mmHg) and an end-diastolic velocity of 1.8 m/s (gradient 13 mmHg). Calculations: PAP_m = 43 mmHg (33 + 10), PAP_d = 23 mmHg (13 + 10), PAP_s = 83 mmHg [(3 × 43) − (2 × 23)] (estimating right arterial pressure as 10 mmHg). (c) Mid-systolic notch of the pulmonary ejection flow (arrow). (d) Lengthening of the pre-ejection time (PET) of the pulmonary flow (PET = 120 ms, ejection time (ET) = 270 ms, PET/ET = 0.44). AO, aorta; PAP_d, PAP_m, PAP_s, diastolic, mean and systolic pulmonary arterial pressures.

> **Box 10.3   Pitfalls in the evaluation of pulmonary pressures when using echo Doppler on the basis of the pulmonary regurgitation (PR) flow**
>
> **Technical pitfalls**
> - Undetectable PR
> - Weak Doppler signal
> - Failure to average the PR velocities
>
> **Diagnostic pitfalls**
> - Errors in the estimation of the right ventricular diastolic pressure
> - Modifications in the morphology of the PR flow (massive PR, dip–plateau)
> - Associated tricuspid stenosis

ary trunk, incomplete detection of the PR in 2D colour Doppler, difficulties of alignment with the small PR jet in continuous Doppler).

Another technical pitfall arises when there is a weak Doppler signal, which largely cannot be analysed using continuous Doppler because:

- the spectral envelope of the PR is poorly defined (incorrect adjustment of the ultrasound machine, poor alignment of the Doppler beam and the PR jet)
- the PR is difficult to explore (eccentric or multiple jets).

In order to avoid these pitfalls, it is necessary to use multiple projections in continuous Doppler: lower left parasternal view, in order to improve the verticalization of the pulmonary orifice, and the subcostal view centred on the trunk of the pulmonary artery.

Finally, as with TR, an average vaue taken over several cardiac cycles may be indispensable when there is wide respiratory variation in the PR curve. However, when there is atrial fibrillation, the measurement of the PR is difficult, even when several values are averaged.

Diagnostic pitfalls

The principal diagnostic pitfall arises from the imprecision of the estimated right ventricular end-diastolic pressure (RVEDP), which is generally evaluated empirically at 10 mmHg. In practice, the right ventricular diastolic pressure is assimilated into the RAP in the absence of tricuspid stenosis. If the potential error caused by the estimation of the RAP for TR is compared with that due to the estimation of the RVEDP in PR, the risk of error is far greater in the latter case, as the RVEDP accounts for about 50% of the value in the calculation of the diastolic PAP, and only 25% of that of the systolic PAP. In fact, under-estimation of the diastolic PAP is common in cases of an elevated RVEDP.

Another diagnostic pitfall is linked to the modifications of the morphology of the PR flow in continuous Doppler, which are observed under certain circumstances:

- annulment of the PR velocity during end-diastole in massive PR

- annulment of the PR velocity during mid-diastole in the case of right ventricular dip–plateau (see Table 7.11 and Fig. 7.28).

Study of the pulmonary ejection flow
The study of the pulmonary ejection flow, which is carried out using pulsed Doppler, may be done in the absence of right valve leaks. In cases of PAHT, the modifications of the pulmonary ejection flow relate to:

- the morphology of the ejection flow
- the systolic intervals (acceleration time, pre-ejection time and pulmonary ejection time).

Morphologically, in place of its usual symmetrical form with a mid-systolic velocity peak, the pulmonary ejection flow may be altered in two ways:

- It becomes triangular, with an earlier peak during systole in cases of moderate PAHT.
- It shows an early systolic peak and a mid-systolic notch (in the deceleration phase) in cases of severe PAHT (Figs. 10.6(c) and 10.7). This mid-systolic notch is due to:
  - the increased pulmonary arterial rigidity, which is a source of reflected pressure waves that tend to close the sigmoid valves
  - a dilatation of the pulmonary trunk, often associated with PAHT, especially severe PAHT, which creates turbulence that can disrupt the permanent opening of the sigmoid valves during systole.

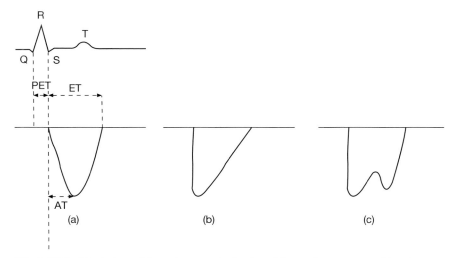

Figure 10.7 Morphology of the pulmonary ejection flow: (a) normal appearance; (b) early peak (moderate pumonary arterial hypertension (PAHT)); (c) mid-systolic notch (severe PAHT). AT, acceleration time; ET, ejection time; PET, pre-ejection time.

Quantitatively, in cases of PAHT the following may be observed:

- lengthening of the pre-ejection time (PET) measured between the beginning of the QRS complex of the electrocardiogram (ECG) and the beginning of the pulmonary flow with a PET/ejection time ratio of > 0.35 (see Fig. 10.6(d))
- lengthening of the acceleration time (AT) measured between the beginning of the flow and the peak of the pulmonary flow with a TA/PET ratio of < 0.36.

In practice, an of AT < 100 ms makes it possible to conclude a mean PAP of > 20 mmHg (see Box 10.1).

The pitfalls relating to the analysis of the pulmonary ejection flow are summarized in Box 10.4. In fact, the parameters calculated using the pulmonary ejection flow depend on:

- the haemodynamic factors (pressures and pulmonary arterial resistances, right ventricular function, cardiac output)
- the Doppler measurement site (pulmonary orifice, infundibulum or pulmonary trunk).

Finally, the idiopathic dilatation of the pulmonary artery may lead to a mid-systolic notch in the pulmonary ejection flow that is independent of any PAHT.

Study of the left-to-right shunt flows

The study of the left-to-right shunt flows enables the calculation of the systolic PAP when there is an interventricular communication or arterial canal (see Box 10.1). The pitfalls when calculating the pulmonary pressures on the basis of the interventricular communication flows are summarized in Box 10.5.

DIFFERENTIAL DIAGNOSIS BETWEEN PRE- AND POSTCAPILLARY PULMONARY ARTERIAL HYPERTENSION

Doppler analysis of the left ventricular filling flows makes it possible to determine the pre- or postcapillary nature of the PAHT. The arguments in favour of a postcapillary PAHT are summarized in Box 10.6.

Box 10.4   Pitfalls in evaluating the pulmonary pressures when using echo Doppler and the pulmonary ejection flow

Technical pitfalls
- Poor spectrum quality rendering the spectrum unanalysable
- Failure to standardize the position of the Doppler measurement volume

Diagnostic pitfalls
- Multiplicity of factors impinging on the parameters of the pulmonary ejection flow
- Idiopathic dilatation of the pulmonary artery

Box 10.5   Pitfalls in the evaluation of the pulmonary pressures when using echo Doppler in cases of interventricular communication

- Poor visualization of the anatomical location of the septal defect
- Complex trajectory of the interventricular communication flow
- Incorrect alignment of the Doppler beam with the interventricular communication flow
- Aortic stenosis or stenosis of the subclavian artery (making it impossible to assimilate the systolic arterial pressure into the left ventricular systolic pressure)
- Associated pulmonary stenosis (making it impossible to assimilate the systolic PAP into the right ventricular systolic pressure)

Box 10.6   Signs indicating postcapillary pulmonary arterial hypertension

- Left heart cardiopathy
- Doppler signs:
    - hypernormal mitral flow: E/A > 2, DT < 130 ms
    - pulmonary venous flow: PAd > MAd
    - mitral propagation velocity < 45 cm/s
    - early diastolic displacement velocity of the mitral annulus < 8 cm/s

DT, deceleration time; MAd, duration of the mitral A wave; PAd, duration of the A wave of pulmonary venous flow.

These are principally Doppler signs suggesting an elevation in left ventricular end-diastolic pressure (> 15 mmHg) characterized by:

- a hypernormal appearance of the mitral flow
- a lengthening of left atrial systole at the level of the pulmonary venous flow
- a marked reduction in the mitral propagation velocity (colour M-mode) and of the mitral annular velocity during early diastole (Doppler tissue imaging).

However, the analysis of these Doppler signs does not make it possible actually to quantify the postcapillary pressures in cases of PAHT. On the other hand, for a given patient, following the Doppler parameters makes it possible to survey the variations in filling pressure, and therefore to assess indirectly the capillary pressure. This advantageous approach nevertheless requires the presence of a sinus rhythm and an effective atrial systole.

INTERPRETATION OF THE VALUES OF THE PULMONARY ARTERIAL PRESSURE

The reliability of the measurement of PAPs when using Doppler imaging is widely acknowledged. The normal resting values are considered to be:

- a systolic PAP < 35 mmHg

- a diastolic PAP < 15 mmHg
- a mean PAP < 25 mmHg.

While a standard estimated error of ± 7 mmHg may be ignored for a systolic PAP of the order of 35 mmHg, it is difficult to do so for a diastolic PAP of the order of 15 mmHg, and thus the precision of the latter measurement is less. In practice, systolic PAP values of > 50 mmHg are always pathological. However, the interpretation of values between 35 and 45 mmHg is sometimes difficult, and the following factors must be taken into account:

- the patient's age
- the patient's body mass
- associated pathology.

The patient's age is one of the most important factors. The threshold of a normal systolic PAP in patients over 60 years old is close to 40 mmHg, while over the age of 70 years this threshold is around 45 mmHg. Obesity or systemic arterial hypertension are also parameters that may modify the PAP reference values in a given patient.

In practice, a systolic PAP > 60 mmHg at rest always points to marked PAHT. However, the coherence of the PAP values with the rest of the clinical presentation and echocardiographic data should be verified systematically.

With regard to the interpretation of the pulmonary pressures during stress echocardiography, the threshold for a normal systolic PAP is 54 mmHg in patients aged under 40 years and 70 mmHg for patients aged over 70 years.

11

Thoracic aorta

The prevalence of aortic pathology is steadily increasing as a result of:

- the ageing population, because ageing is accompanied by progressive modifications of the cardiovascular system
- the high incidence of arterial hypertension, which increases progressively with age
- a better understanding of aortic pathology due to improvements in diagnostic techniques.

Transoesophageal echocardiography (TEE) has become a complementary technique to transthoracic echocardiography (TTE), and one that is almost indispensable in studying aortic pathologies such as dissection, haematoma, aneurysm and atheroma of the thoracic aorta.

However, despite significant progress in echo Doppler technology, the diversity of the aetiologies and the complexity of the aortic lesions are sometimes bewildering to the echocardiographer.

AORTIC DISSECTION

Aortic dissection is a medico-surgical emergency that requires a precise diagnosis as early as possible.

TEE is a highly effective first-line diagnostic method, and is easily carried out at the patient's bedside. It can be used to explore almost the entire thoracic aorta. However, it requires an experienced echocardiographer and, in case of any doubt, recourse to another imaging technique. In cardiological practice, TEE is always preceded by TTE, which may already suggest the diagnosis.

The limitations and pitfalls of TEE relate to:

- the identification of the aortic dissection
- the precise location of the dissection
- the detection of complications associated with the dissection.

Given the clinical gravity of aortic dissection, and particularly in emergency cases, good familiarity with these pitfalls is crucial.

Pitfalls when diagnosing dissection
These pitfalls are due to:

- reduced specificity of the echocardiographic signs of dissection

- the sometimes difficult distinction between the true and false lumen
- imprecise visualization of the dissection point of entry.

Specificity of the echocardiographic signs

The echocardiographic diagnosis of aortic dissection is based on the visualization of the mobile intimal flap, floating between the true and false lumen (Figs 11.1 and 11.2).

The identification of this intimal flap is pathognomonic for the diagnosis of dissection, but there are diagnostic pitfalls of overdiagnosis (false-positive results) and underdiagnosis (false-negative results), which should be guarded against.

Overdiagnosis of aortic dissection

False-positive diagnoses of aortic dissection (Box 11.1) are dominated by:

- so-called linear artefacts located in the aortic lumen and simulating an intimal flap (Fig. 11.3)
- intra-aortic reverberations from thick aortic walls or a calcified aortic ring may be falsely interpreted as a dissection.

Linear artefacts, which are located principally on the ascending aorta, are frequently observed in monoplanar TEE. The use of multiplanar TEE has reduced the incidence of these aretefacts, but has not resolved the problem: the arte-

---

Box 11.1   Causes of false-positive diagnosis of aortic dissection when using TEE

- Ultrasound artefacts (linear or mirrored)
- Ultrasound reverberations due to thickened aortic walls, a calcified aortic annulus or a mediastinal extracardiac structure (haematoma, abscess, tumour, fat)
- Annular ectasia of the aorta with abnormally long aortic sigmoid valves, which may be confused with an intimal flap
- An aneurysm of the descending thoracic aorta, with a mural thrombus simulating a thrombotic false lumen
- A false aortic aneurysm, which may give the appearance of a localized pseudodissection
- An isthmic rupture
- An abscess of the aortic cuff
- A detached atheromatous plaque, called a 'floating' plaque, within the aortic lumen
- An intra-aortic clapper-shaped thrombus, sometimes floating
- A pleural effusion
- A vascular superposition (innominate venous trunk, hemizygotic vein)
- Theile transverse sinus
- The spinal canal

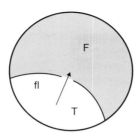

Figure 11.1 Schematic appearance of an aortic dissection with a true lumen (T), false lumen (F), intimal flap (fl) and entry point (arrow). Transverse view of the aorta.

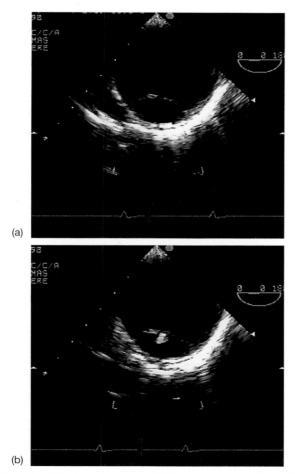

Figure 11.2 Dissection of the thoracic aorta in TEE (transverse view). (a) Intimal flap with the entry point separating the aortic lumen into two channels. (b) Dissection entry point detected using colour Doppler.

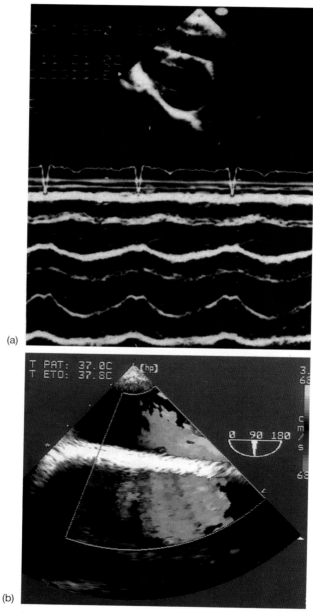

(a)

(b)

Figure 11.3   Artefactual images of aortic dissection in TEE. (a) Linear artefacts within the ascending aorta; anterior artefact with amplitude and movement double that of the posterior wall of the aorta. (b) Mirror-image-type artefact at the level of the descending thoracic aorta observed in colour Doppler. (Images by Prof. R. Roudaut.)

factual images are often found in different planes. Linear artefacts stem from multiple reflections of the ultrasound off the walls of the left atrium in particular. They arise in the presence of a wide aorta, with a diameter greater than that of the left atrium, with the ultrasound probe at a distance equal to or double the atrial diameter (Fig. 11.4). In fact, an aortic diameter of > 50 mm and a left atrium/ aorta ratio of < 0.6 are excellent predictive factors for the creation of artefacts.

Three principal types of artefact have been described that are due to the reflection of the ultrasound from either the posterior wall of the left atrium (type A), the posterior wall of the right pulmonary artery (type C) or the interaction between the two (type B). Type A linear artefacts, due to the reflection by the aorta/left atrium interface, are the most common. They may be easily identified by their particular echocardiographic appearance, especially when using M-mode (Box 11.2), which makes it possible to avoid an erroneous diagnosis of aortic dissection.

Artefactual images may also be encountered at the level of the descending thoracic aorta. The interpretation of these images is generally easier. Generally, the artefacts are mirror images of the descending thoracic aorta, which may be seen on TEE in cases of tortuous aorta in particular. The artefacts are probably linked to multiple reflections between the aorta and the adjacent pleuropulmonary space, producing a split image of the aortic lumen, with the Doppler flow present in the true lumen and in the mirror image (see Fig. 11.3).

Normal anatomical structures may also give rise to images that can deceive inexperienced observers, such as the innominate venous trunk or a small calibre blood vessel that runs parallel to the horizontal aorta. However, the flow in this vessel when examined using Doppler is of the venous type. Likewise, the hemizygotic vein, which has a parallel trajectory to the descending thoracic aorta, may lead to a false splitting of the aortic lumen, as may the Theile transverse sinus (Fig. 11.5). These anatomical pitfalls are easily avoided with experience.

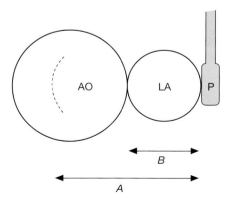

Figure 11.4 Creation of a type A linear artefact in the ascending aorta (AO) that is larger than the left atrium (LA). The artefact (dashed line) is projected into the aortic lumen at a distance equal to or double the atrial diameter ($A = 2B$). P, ultrasound probe.

Box 11.2   Echocardiographic signs that suggest an ultrasound artefact simulating aortic dissection

- Linear artefactual images that are > 2.5 mm thick, of low mobility and have blurred contours

- The displacement of the artefact parallels that of the posterior wall of the aorta

- The distance between the posterior wall of the ascending aorta and the artefact is identical to the distance between the probe and the posterior wall of the aorta

- The absence of broad oscillations of the artefact (as opposed to a highly mobile dissection flap, with expansion of the true lumen during systole)

- The absence of an identifiable entry point to the dissection (no aliasing phenomenon in colour Doppler, which may indicate the existence of an entry point)

- The absence of a double lumen appearance, with different flow velocities in pulsed and colour Doppler (identical velocities on either part of the artefact)

- The possible continuation of the artefact beyond the aortic walls

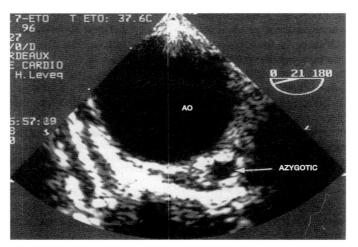

Figure 11.5   Azygotic vein creating a pseudo-splitting of the descending thoracic aorta (AO), as visualized in TEE. (Image by Prof. R. Roudaut.)

Finally, one particular diagnostic pitfall is worthy of emphasis. A traumatic rupture of the aorta at the isthmic level may wrongly suggest a diagnosis of aortic dissection. The TEE signs that make it possible to distinguish between these two conditions are summarized in Table 11.1.

Underdiagnosis of aortic dissection

False-negative diagnoses of aortic dissection (Box 11.3) are much less common than false-positive ones, and occur principally in highly localized forms of dissection, or where a complete thrombosis of the false lumen makes identification of the intimal flap extremely difficult.

Table 11.1 Differential diagnosis between an isthmic rupture of the aorta and an aortic dissection as visualized in TEE

	Isthmic rupture	Aortic dissection
Location of the lesion	Isthmus	Variable
Isthmic contours	Asymmetrical	Symmetrical
Intimal–medial flap (longitudinal cross-section)	Medial flap: thick, highly mobile, perpendicular to the isthmus walls	Intimal flap: thin, less mobile, parallel to the aortic walls
Entry point	Absent	Present
Blood velocities	Similar on either side of the flap	Different in each lumen
Thrombus	Absent	Possible in the false lumen
Mediastinal haematoma	Present	Absent

Box 11.3 Causes of false-negative diagnosis of aortic dissection when using TEE

- Poor echocardiographic imaging
- Type A dissections affecting the ascending aorta in the 'blind zone'
- Low, type B dissections located at the junction of the thoracic aorta and the abdominal aorta
- A complete thrombosis of the false lumen, masking the intimal flap
- Very low echogenicity of the intimal flap
- A very narrow false lumen
- A retrograde extension of the dissection with thrombosis of the false lumen
- An intramural haematoma (incipient dissection)

Finally, an aortic intramural haematoma may mask an incipient aortic dissection. Moreover, the differential diagnosis between intramural haematoma and aortic dissection with early and complete thrombosis of the false lumen may be difficult in certain cases. The classical echocardiographic signs indicating an aortic haematoma are summarized in Box 11.4.

Aortic intramural haematoma

Aortic intramural haematoma is defined as a spontaneous and localized intramural haemorrhage (Fig. 11.6). It is most commonly found in the descending thoracic aorta. The intramural haematoma develops in the media of the aortic wall, the essential difference between this and classical dissection being the absence of an intimal tear. The spontaneous evolution of the haematoma, meanwhile, is highly variable: stabilization, dissection, rupture, but also progressive regression.

TEE is the best choice of examination for identifying an aortic intramural haematoma (Fig. 11.7). Its only limitation is in the area of the aortic arch, where a small, highly localized haematoma may go unnoticed.

Box 11.4   Echocardiographic signs of an aortic haematoma

- Localized thickening of the aortic wall, crescent-shaped or circumferential, > 7 mm
- Deformation of the aortic lumen, with an increased external diameter of the aorta
- Centroluminal backflow of the intimal calcifications
- Variable structural echogenicity (plain or 'stippled' appearance of a fresh or organized haematoma, 'cystic' empty appearance in the case of liquefaction)
- Enlargement of the distance between the oesophagus and the descending thoracic aortic lumen
- Absence of an entry point, intimal flap and false lumen
- Signs of blood extravasation signifying the external rupture of the haematoma (haemomediastinum, haemothorax)

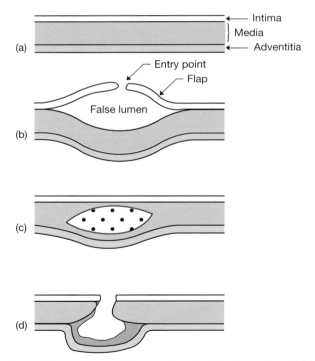

Figure 11.6   Schematic appearance of the normal and pathological aortic wall: (a) three tunica of the normal aortic wall; (b) subintimal dissection; (c) fresh intramedial haematoma; (d) thrombotic false subadventitial aneurysm.

False-positive diagnoses are indicated by:

- a localized thrombotic dissection
- a mural thrombus on an aneurysmal aorta
- a significant atheromatous thickening.

Distinction between the true and false lumen

The echocardiographic differentiation between the true and false lumen is based on several TEE criteria (Box 11.5). Familiarity with these criteria is vital, as the size of the false lumen and its circulatory character are important prognostic elements. In fact, the (external) false lumen, created by the irruption of

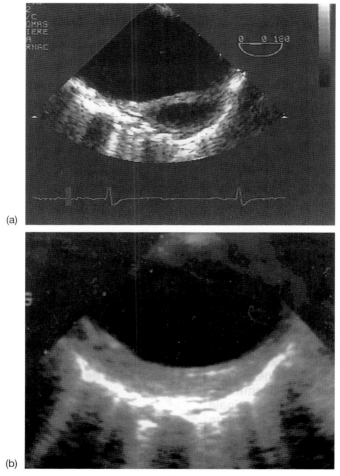

(a)

(b)

Figure 11.7   Aortic intramural haematoma (in TEE) with cystic appearance (a) and full crescent-shaped appearance (b). (Images by Dr. J.-Ph. Baguet.)

> **Box 11.5 Criteria for distinguishing between the true and false lumen when using TEE**
>
> - Channel size: false lumen larger than true lumen
> - Systolic movement of the flap: expansion towards the false lumen
> - Appearance of the flow through the entry point: directed from the true lumen towards the false lumen
> - Blood circulation: faster in the true lumen

blood into the split aortic wall, is generally wider than the (internal) true lumen. The velocity of the flow circulating in the true lumen is higher than that in the false lumen (Fig. 11.8). However, the blood flow may be very slow within the false lumen and seen on the image as a spontaneous contrast effect (see page 154). In certain favourable cases, a complete thrombosis of the false lumen occurs, cutting off circulation. This thrombosis is frequent in chronic forms of dissection and dissections of the descending thoracic aorta. However, it is not uncommon in acute dissections and, if it damages the ascending aorta or the aortic arch, it is necessary to consider the possibility of a retrograde dissection.

Identification of the entry point

The two channels separated by the intimal flap communicate by means of the entry point, which corresponds to the tear in the intima. It is possible to identify this tear, which determines the surgery, using two-dimensional (2D) colour Doppler (see Figs. 11.2 and 11.8). Classically, the narrow and aliased colour jet passes through the entry point from the true lumen into the false lumen during systole. The diagnostic pitfalls to be aware of are:

- The absence of an entry point at the level of the dissected ascending aorta. In this case, it is necessary to seek the intimal rupture at the level of the horizontal aorta or the aortic isthmus (retrograde type dissection).
- The presence of multiple entry points.
- The existence of the entry orifice and exit orifice (called the re-entry orifice), enabling the blood to return to the aortic lumen from the false lumen.
- The bidirectional systolodiastolic appearance of the flow between the two channels. This situation is most commonly encountered when there is a wide intimal laceration.

Pitfalls when localizing the dissection

TEE can be used to determine the location and extent of the dissection by means of a systematic sweeping of the different aortic segments. This analysis is made easier by the use of multiplanar TEE probes, which enable an almost complete exploration of the thoracic aorta, in particular the ascending part, which is expulsed over 8–10 cm in a longitudinal plane.

The pitfalls when using TEE to locate a dissection may relate to:

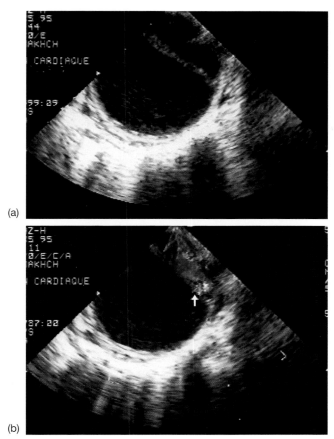

Figure 11.8 Aortic dissection in TTE (transverse view). Blood flow visualized using colour Doppler in the true lumen. The entry point of the dissection is identified in blue (arrow in (b)). Spontaneous contrast is present in the false lumen.

- A small upper part of the ascending aorta, which is practically inaccessible using monoplanar TEE (blind zone) due to the interposition of the trachea between the probe and the aorta. In fact, dissections strictly limited to this portion of the aorta are very much the exception.
- Anteretrograde and/or retrograde extension of the dissection.
- The circumferential form of the dissection.
- The longitudinal and/or transverse propagation of the dissection.
- Multiple dissections layered over the aorta (e.g. localized dissection of the ascending aorta associated with a dissection of the descending aorta).
- Peripheral dissections (progression of the dissection in the collateral arteries of the aorta: carotid, renal, iliac, digestive).

These pitfalls may be avoided by carrying out a precise and complete examination of the aortic lesions using multiplanar TEE.

Pitfalls relating to the complications of dissection

During the examination, the echocardiographer must strive to uncover any possible complications of the aortic dissection, which might aggravate the prognosis of the condition and, most importantly, require specific surgery.

The echocardiographic pitfalls relate to the precise examination of the different complications, such as:

- progressive distension of the aorta, increasing the risk of late wall rupture
- aortic regurgitation, whereby the mechanism must be specified (distension of the annulus, prolapse or hooding of one or more sigmoid valves secondary to the rupture of a commissure due to the dissection process, invagination of the intimal flap in the normal aortic sigmoid valves)
- extension of the dissection into the coronary artery
- a pericardial effusion indicating a tear in the ascending aorta in the pericardium
- periaortic or mediastinal haematoma
- the appearance of a false aneurysm at the level of an anastomosis of a vascular prosthesis.

These potential complications of dissection may be missed during a rapid echocardiographic examination, and thus it is important to take time to examine carefully the whole of the aorta and the adjacent structures, or even to repeat the TEE examination if doubt remains.

In conclusion, the limitations and pitfalls of echocardiographic examination discussed above should not in any way call into question the significant diagnostic benefits of TEE in the detection of aortic dissections. In fact, a careful and precise analysis of the characteristics of the artefactual echoes and the ratios between the aorta and the neighbouring structures, as well as the use of different TEE planes coupled with Doppler, enables mistaken interpretations of the diagnosis to be avoided, and the specificity of the TEE diagnoses of aortic dissections to be increased.

AORTIC ANEURYSMS

Aortic aneurysms appear on the echocardiographic image as a localized dilatation of the aorta with a loss of parallelism of its walls. The normal diameter values of the thoracic aorta according to the segment under consideration are summarized in Fig. 11.9.

TEE makes it possible to specify the size, type (sacciform or fusiform) and the location of aneurysms of the thoracic aorta. The diagnostic pitfalls relate to:

- An often unrecognized intra-aneurysmal thrombosis.
- The sometimes very difficult differential diagnosis between a thrombotic fusiform aneurysm and thrombosis of the false lumen of an aortic dissection.
- Annular ectasia of the ascending aorta, with abnormally long aortic sigmoid valves, which may simulate the intimal flap.
- Aneurysm of the sinus of Valsalva creating a fissure in the right chambers (Fig. 11.10).

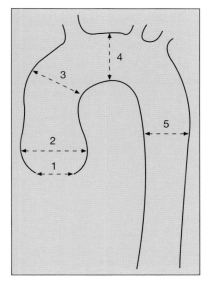

Segment	Location	Diameter (cm)
1	Aortic annulus	1.9 ± 0.2
2	Sinus of Valsalva	2.8 ± 0.3
3	Ascending aorta	2.6 ± 0.3
4	Horizontal aorta	2.4 ± 0.2
5	Descending aorta	1.7 ± 0.3

Figure 11.9 Echocardiographic measurements of the diameter of the thoracic aorta (average values in centimetres) in the normal adult.

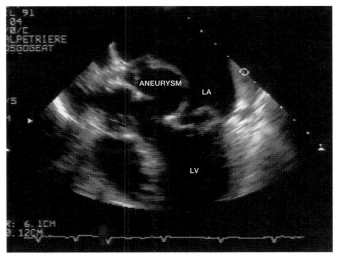

Figure 11.10 Aneurysm of the posterior sinus of Valsalva as seen in TEE. LA, left atrium; LV, left ventricle.

- A false aneurysm at the level of the aortic isthmus. This is generally a post-traumatic sacciform aneurysm communicating with the native aorta by means of a more or less broad neck, and often presenting a thrombus that more or less fills the aneurysm (see Fig. 11.6).

- Aneurysmal fissure of the pericardium, which has the same echocardiographic signs as a pericardial effusion.
- Progressive evolution of the aneurysm towards the aortic dissection (dissecting aneurysm).

A lack of familiarity with these particular situations may render interpretation of the TEE examination difficult.

AORTIC ATHEROMA

TEE can be used to easily detect atheromatous plaques of the thoracic aorta and to determine their location and appearance (Figs 11.11 and 11.12).

The possible pitfalls when diagnosing aortic atheroma relate in particular to:

- the precise location of the plaques at the level of the different aortic segments
- the detailed evaluation of the shape of the plaques (smooth, irregular, uneven, protrusive) and their echo structure (homogeneous or heterogeneous)
- the detection of a sessile or pedunculated mobile thrombus associated with the plaque
- the identification of the pedunculated mobile atheromatous elements, known as intra-aortic debris

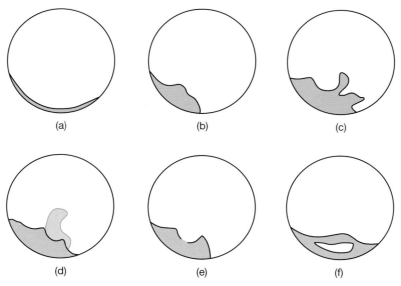

Figure 11.11 Morphological forms of atheromatous lesions identifiable using TEE (transverse aortic view): (a) isolated regular thickening of the intima; (b) smooth, homogeneous, simple atheromatous plaque; (c) uneven, heterogeneous, pedunculated plaque; (d) plaque complicated by a superadded thrombus; (e) ulcerated plaque complicated by an intimal rupture; (f) a haematoma formed in the plaque.

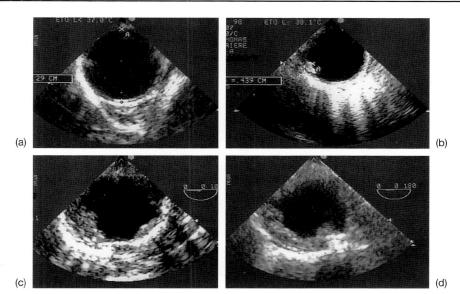

Figure 11.12   Examples of aortic atheroma viewed in TEE (transverse cross-sections of the thoracic aorta): (a) discrete regular thickening of the aortic intima; (b) isolated, partially detached atheromatous plaque, 4.4 mm thick; (c) ulcerated, irregular, thick, broad aortic atheroma, with wall calcifications; (d) voluminous aortic atheroma complicated by a mobile thrombus located on the plaque.

- the formation of a haematoma beneath the plaque, which may evolve towards the aortic dissection.

Familiarity with these pitfalls makes it possible to avoid mistaken interpretation of the examination, and to identify complex plaques with mobile elements risking peripheral embolisms.

Finally, it is important always to undertake an 'echocardiographic once-over' of the abdominal aorta, as the fortuitous discovery of an aortic aneurysm is actually not uncommon.

This is the last 'echocardiographic pitfall' covered in this work, and it is of major diagnostic importance, both for the doctor and the patient.

Bibliography

ABERGEL E. Détection et quantification de l'hypertension artérielle pulmonaire. *Réalités Cardiologiques* 1997; **120**: 6–8.

ABERGEL E., TASE M., BOHLENDER J. et al. Which definition for echocardiographic left ventricular hypertrophy? *Am. J. Cardiol.* 1995; **75**: 489–502.

ABERGEL E., MENARD J. L'échocardiographie chez l'hypertendu: comment, pourquoi et pour qui? *Act. Méd. Int.* 1997; **2**: 85–92

ACAR Ch. et al. Intégrale: insuffisance mitrale. *Cardiologie Pratique* 2002; 616–617.

APPELBE A.F., WALKER P.C., YEOH J.K. et al. Clinical significance and origin of artefacts in transoesophageal echocardiography of the thoracic aorta. *J. Am. Coll. Cardiol.* 1993; **21**: 754–760.

APPLETON C.P., GALLONAY J.M., GONZALEZ M.S. et al. Estimation of left ventricular filling pressures using two-dimensional and Doppler echocardiography in adult patients with cardiac disease. *J. Am. Coll. Cardiol.* 1993; **22**: 1972–1982.

APPLETON C.P., HATLE L.K., POPP R.L. Relation of transmitral flow velocity patterns to left ventricular diastolic function: new insight from a combined hemodynamic and Doppler echocardiographic study. *J. Am. Coll. Cardiol.* 1988; **12**: 426–440.

Arch. Mal. Cœur Prat. 1997; **56**: 17–19.

ARQUES S. Pressions de remplissage en échocardiographie Doppler. *Arch. Mal. Cœur Prat.* 2004; **128**: 13–15.

BARLOW J.B., BOSMAN C.K. Aneurysmal protusion of the posterior leaflet of the mitral valve: an ausculatory echocardiographic syndrome. *Am. Heart J.* 1966; **71**: 166–178.

BAUER F. Fonction systolique conservée et flux transmitral restrictif: péricarde ou myocarde? *Arch. Mal. Cœur Prat.* 2004; **129**: 13–14.

BAUMGARTNER H., STEFENELLI T. Overestimation of catheter gradients by Doppler ultrasound in patients with aortic stenosis: a predictable manifestation of pressure recovery. *J. Am. Coll. Cardiol.* 1999; **33**: 1655–1661.

BENNIS A. Péricardite chronique constrictive. Apport de l'écho-Doppler. *Arch. Med. Cœur Prat.* 1998; **60**: 15–17.

BENNIS A., CHRAIBI S., SOULAMI S. et al. Dissection de l'aorte. Intérêt de l'échocardiographie transœsophagienne. *Cardiologie Pratique* 1997; **397**: 3–7.

BENSAÏD J. et al. Insuffisance mitrale dégénérative. *Cardiologie Pratique* 2000; **510/511**: 11–18.

BERREBI A. Évaluation échographique (ETT et ETO) de la faisabilité d'une plastie mitrale. *Cardiologie Pratique* 2003; **635**: 9–12.

BOCHET E., ASSAYA G.P., BENAMER H. et al. Diagnostic des dissections aortiques en ETO. Attention aux images pièges. *Cardiologie Pratique* 1996; **387**.

BRAUNWALD E. *Heart Diseases. A Textbook of Cardiovascular Medicine*, 5th edn. Saunders, Philadelphia, 1997, pp. 1154–1170.

BROCHET E. Apport de l'échographie transœsophagienne dans la pathologie de l'aorte. *Cardioscopie* 1996; **39**: 63–81.

BROCHET E. Écho-Doppler cardiaque dans l'infarctus du myocarde. *Cardiologie Pratique* 2002; **627**: 4–5.

BRUNITZ J.F. Critères d'évaluation des zones ventriculaires gauches infarcies et quantification. *Réalités Cardiologiques* 1995; **82**: 32–39.

Cardiologie Pratique 1988; **85**: 1–4.

CHARRON Ph. Cardiomyopathie hypertrophique: quoi de neuf? *Cardiologie Pratique* 2003; **640**: 14–16.

CHARRON Ph. Les myocardiopathies restrictives. *La Lettre du Cardiologue* 1999; **312**: 21–29.

CHAUVEL C. Analyse de la fonction ventriculaire gauche dans les cardiopathies ischémiques. *Cardiologie Pratique* 2002; **612**: 1–3.

CHAUVEL C. Étude de la fonction diastolique ventriculaire gauche par échocardiographie Doppler. *Cardiologie Pratique* 1997; **420**: 1–3.

CHAUVEL C., ABERGEL E., COHEN A. Hypertrophie ventriculaire gauche: physiologique et pathologique? *Le Cardiologue* 2002; **256**: 27–34.

CHAUVEL C., DEHANT P., BOGINO E. Évaluation écho-Doppler des insuffisances aortiques. *Cardiologie Pratique* 1999, **476**: 6–9.

COHEN A. Échocardiographie transœsophagienne et embolie artérielle. *Cardiologie Pratique* 1994; **292**: 5–14.

COHEN A., CHAUVEL C. et al. *Échocardiographie de Stress*. Estem, Paris, 1996.

COHEN A., TZOURIO C., AMARENCO P. Évaluation de l'athérosclérose aortique par échocardiographie transœsophagienne. Implications pronostiques. *Arch. Mal. Coeur* 1997; **90**(II): 11–23.

CORMIER B. Les nouveaux critères diagnostiques du prolapsus valvulaire mitral. *Réalités Cardiologiques* 2000; **156**: 29–30.

CORMIER B., DIEBOLD B., GUERET P. et al. L'échographie dans le diagnostic de l'endocardite infectieuse: fiabilité et limites. *Arch. Mal. Coeur* 1993; **86**: 1819–1823.

COSSON S., ADAMS C., LAMISSE N., COHEN A. Échocardiographie de stress et rétrécissement mitral. *Réalités Cardiologiques* 2003; **187**: 31–37.

DE MARIA A.N., WISENBAUGH T.N., SMITH M.D. et al. Doppler echocardiographic evaluation of diastolic dysfunction. *Circulation* 1991; **84**(Suppl. I): 288–295.

DE MARIA R., DÜRRIEMAN N., RISPALI P. et al. Endocardites fongiques. *Arch. Mal. Cœur Prat.* 2001; **97**: 29–30.

DEHANT P. Anatomie échographique de la valve mitrale. *Cardiologie Pratique* 1997; **425**: 7–9.

DELAHAYE F. et al. Intégrale: endocardite infectieuse de l'adulte. *Cardiologie Pratique* 2001; 556.

DENIS B. Comment mesurer le débit cardiaque? *Cardiologie Pratique* 1995; **315**: 1–4.

DERUMEAUX G. Quels indices utiliser en Doppler tissulaire? *Arch. Mal. Cœur.* 2003; **96**(V): 9–14.

DERUMEAUX G., ELTCHANINOFF H., LETAC B. Rétrécissement mitral: critères écho-Doppler de sévérité. *Cardioscopie* 1993; **16**: 289–293.

DEVEREUX R.P., KOREN M.J., DE SIMONE G. et al. Left ventricular mass as a measure of preclinical hypertensive disease. *Am. Heart J.* 1992; **5**: 175–181.

DIB J.C. Quantification d'une insuffisance mitrale en écho-Doppler cardiaque. *Et. Eval. Cardiovasc.* 1996; **3**: 93–102.

DIB J.C. Quantification d'une sténose aortique en écho-Doppler. *Cardiologie Pratique* 1990; **364**: 11–13.

DIB J.C., ABERGEL E., ROVANI C. et al. The age of the patient should be taken account when interpretating Doppler assessed pulmonary artery pressures. *J. Am Soc. Echocardiogr.* 1997; **10**: 72–73.

DORMAGEN V. Comment diagnostiquer une tamponnade? *Réalités Cardiologiques* 1994; **68**: 22–25.

DUBOURG O. Rupture traumatique de l'aorte. *Cardiologie Pratique* 1997; **402**: 11.

DUBOURG O., BOURDARIAS J.-P. Exploration échographique Doppler des myocardiopathies. *Arch. Mal. Coeur* 1996; **89**(II): 39–45.

DUBOURG O., VINSONNEAU Ch. Analyse échographique du cœur droit. *Cardiologie Pratique* 2000; **541**:18–22.

DUVAL A.M. Critères d'évaluation des HTAP. *Réalités Cardiologiques* 1996; **94**: 45–49.

FARCOT J.C. *Comprendre l'Echocardiographie*. MSD Médicales, Paris, 1986.

FEIGENBAUM H. *Echocardiography*. Lea and Febiger, Philadelphia, 1994.

FRANGOS A. Le diagnostic échocardiographique du cœur hypertensif. *Inform. Cardiol.* 1994; **XVIII**(2): 56–59.

GALLET B. Avantages et limites des différentes méthodes d'estimation des pressions artérielles pulmonaires. *Cardiologie Pratique* 1994; **290**: 8–11.

GALLET B. Comment évaluer la fonction diastolique du ventricule gauche par écho-cardiographie Doppler en l'an 2000. *La Lettre du Cardiologue* 2000; **324**: 25–36.

GALLET B. Estimation des pressions de remplissage et des pressions pulmonaires par échocardiographie Doppler. *Cardiologie Pratique* 2004; **684**: 1–5.

GALLET B. Estimation des pressions de remplissage par échocardiographie Doppler. *Arch. Mal. Cœur Prat.* 2003: 5–12.

GALLET B. Évaluation échocardiographique du rétrécissement aortique. Problèmes pratiques et nouveautés. *Cardiologie Pratique* 2001; **580**: 1–4.

GALLET B. Fonction diastolique. *Arch. Mal. Coeur Prat.* 2000; **87**: 25–27.

GALLET B. Modalités pratiques de mesure des paramètres de la fonction diastolique. *Réalités Cardiologiques;* 2002; **175**: 27–31.

GALLET B. Nouveautés dans la quantification du rétrécissement mitral en échocardiographie doppler. *Cardiologie Pratique* 1998; **447**: 10–13.

GALLET B. Quantification de l'insuffisance mitrale en échocardiographie Doppler. *Cardiologie Pratique* 1998; **445**: 1–5.

GARCIA M.J., PALAC R.T., MALENKA D.J. et al. Color M-mode Doppler flow propagation velocity is a relatively preload-independent index of left ventricular filling. *J. Am. Soc. Echocardiogr.* 1999; **12**: 129–137.

GARCIA M.J., THOMAS J.D., KLEIN A.L. New Doppler echocardiographic applications for the study of diastolic function. *J. Am. Coll. Cardiol.* 1998; **32**: 865–875.

GOSSE Ph., GUEZ D., GUERET P. et al. Centralized echocardiogram quality control in a multicenter study of regression of left ventricular hypertrophy in hypertension. *J. Hypertens.* 1998; **16**: 531–535.

GUERET P., BENSAÏD J. L'échocardiographie: instrument d'évaluation quantitative du remodelage ventriculaire. *Arch. Mal. Coeur* 1991; **84**: 21–27.

GUERET P., MONIN J.-L., DUVAL A-M., GAROT J. L'essentiel de 1999 en échocardiographie. *Arch. Mal. Coeur* 2000; **93**(1): 33–41.

GUITI C., DUBOURG O. Diagnostic échographique des myocardiopathies hypertrophiques. *Réalités Cardiologiques* 1997; **106**: 8–11.

HABIB G. Échocardiographie et critères diagnostiques de l'endocardite infectieuse. *Cardiologie Pratique* 2001; **554**: 6–7.

HAGEGE A. Cardiomyopathie hypertrophique. Qu'attend le clinicien de l'échographiste? *Cardiologie Pratique* 2003; **651**: 1–3.

HAGEGE A. Dépistage et explorations des dysfonctions ventriculaires gauches. *La Revue du Praticien* 1998; **48**: 19–22.

HAGEGE A. Échocardiographie 3D temps réel. *La lettre du Cardiologue* 2004; **373**: 27–30.

HAGEGE A. Révision des critères échocardiographiques du prolapsus valvulaire mitral.

HAGEGE A., MIROCHNIK N., GUEROT T C. Reconstructions tridimensionnelles des structures cardiaques par échocardiographie. *Cardinale* 1998; **X**(9): 10–13.

HATLE L.K., APPLETON C.P., POPP R.L. Differenciation of constrictive pericarditis and restrictive cardiomyopathy by Doppler echocardiography. *J. Am. Coll. Cardiol.* 1994; **23**: 154–162.

HEINLE S.K., HALL S.A., BRICKNER E et al. Comparison of vena contracta width by multiplane transoesophageal echocardiography with quantitative Doppler assessment of mitral regurgitation. *Am. J. Cardiol.* 1998; **81**: 175–178.

HERPIN D.L.'échocardiogramme chez l'hypertendu. *Arch. Mal. Cœur* 2000; **91**:19–21.

HOFFMAN P., Kaasprzak J. *Echokardiografia.* Via Medica, Gdansk, 2004.

ISAAZ K., DERUMEAUX G., GARCIA-FERNANDEZ M.A. et al. Le Doppler tissulaire myocardique. *Réalités Cardiologiques* 1999; **139**: 2.

IUNG B. Détection de l'hypertrophie ventriculaire gauche. *Cardiologie Pratique* 1996; **362**: 1–3.

IUNG B. La maladie annulo-ectasiante de l'aorte. *La Lettre du Cardiologue* 2003; **367**: 35–39.

JAMES M., RIPPE B.A., ANGOFF G. et al. Multiple floppy valves: an echocardiographic syndrome. *Am. J. Med.* 1979; **66**: 817–824.

KASPRZAK J.D., SAUSTRI A., ROELANDT J.K. et al. Three dimensional echocardiography of the aorte valve: feasibility, clinical potential and limitations. *Echocardiography* 1998; **15(2)**: 127–138.

KIENY J.R., FAVIER J.P., GRISON D. et al. Le bourrelet septal sous-aortique. À propos de 23 cas. *Ann. Cardiol. Angéiol.* 1985; **35(5)**: 251–256.

KLIMCZAK CH, DROBINSKI G., LASCAULT G. et al. Limites de l'échocardiographie dans le diagnostic du prolapsus valvulaire mitral. *Inform. Cardiol.* 1986; **7–8**: 582–587.

KLIMCZAK Ch. *Échocardiographie Clinique.* Masson, Paris, 2001.

KLIMCZAK Ch. *Échocardiographie de Stress.* Masson, Paris, 1997.

KLIMCZAK Ch. *Échographie Cardiaque du Sujet Âgé.* Acanthe/Masson, Paris, 2000.

KLIMCZAK Ch. *Échographie Cardiaque Transœsophagienne.* Masson, Paris, 2002.

KLIMCZAK Ch., CHEVALLIER P., DROBINSKI G. et al. Difficultés du diagnostic échocardiographique du prolapsus valvulaire mitral. *JEMU* 1986; **3**: 125–133.

LAFITTE S., ROUDANT R. Intérêt de l'échocardiographie dans l'insuffisance cardiaque. *Cardiologie Pratique* 2004; **695**(Suppl.): 14–18.

LAPERCHE T. L'athérome de la crosse aortique. *Abst. Cardiologie* 2004; **393**: 27–29.

LARDOUX H., BOYNARD M., CORMIER B. et al. Contraste spontané intracardiaque et risque embolique. *Arch. Mal. Coeur* 1996; **89**: 451–457.

LAUER M.S., ANDERSON K.M., LARSON M.G. et al. A new method for indexing left ventricular mass for differences in body size. *Am. J. Cardiol.* 1994; **74**: 487–491.

LAURENCEAU J.-L., MALERGUE M.-C. *L'Essentiel sur l'Echocardiographie.* Maloine, Paris, 1980.

LESBRE J.P., RUIZ V. Les abcès para-annulaires. Diagnostic clinique et échographique.

LESBRE J.R., TRIBOUILLOY C., JAUBOURG M.L. et al. Abcès para-annulaires. À propos de 59 cas. Étude multicentrique. *Arch. Mal. Coeur* 1995; **88**: 321–328.

LUTFALLA G. Comment calculer la surface mitrale en imagerie et en Doppler? *Réalités Cardiologiques* 1994; **65**: 18–22.

LUTFALLA G. Comment étudier la fonction systolique et diastolique du ventricule droit en échographie doppler. *Réalités Cardiologiques* 1995; **75**: 17–22.

LUTFALLA G. Comment mesurer la taille des cavités droites en échographie? *Réalités Cardiologiques*, 1995; **74**: 4–11.

LUTFALLA G., RAFFOUL H., DERUMEAUX G. Fonction diastolique à l'écho-Doppler. *Réalités Cardiologiques* 1996; **103**: 7- 24.

MALERGUE M.Ch. Fonction ventriculaire gauche. La valeur prédictive des index écho-Doppler. *Cardinale* 2001, XIII; 10: 32–37.

MIROCHNIK N. Échocardiographie tridimensionnelle dans l'évaluation des valvulopathies. *Cardinale* 2002; **XIV**(5): 26–29.

MIRODE A., TRIBOUILLOY C., MAZOUZ S., LESBRE J.P. Évaluation par écho-Doppler de la sévérité des régurgitations mitrales. *Réalités Cardiologiques* 1994; **58**: 31–36.

MONIN J.L. Hématome intrapariétal aortique. *Cardiologie Pratique* 2004; **688**: 3–5.

MONIN J.L. Rétrécissement aortique calcifié en bas débit. Évaluation, du risque opératoire par échographie dobutamine faible dose. *Cardiologie Pratique* 2002; **606/607**: 6–7.

MONIN J.L. Rétrécissement aortique calcifié. Les pièges de la quantification en écho-Doppler transthoracique. *Cardiologie Pratique* 2003; **658**: 1–4.

MONIN J.L. Utilité clinique de l'écho-dobutamine pour l'évaluation des sténoses aortiques. *Réalités Cardiologiques* 1998; **132**: 15–18.

NAGUEH S.F., MIDDLETON K.J., KOPELEN H.A. et al. Doppler tissue imaging: a non invasive technic for evaluation of left ventricular relaxation and estimation of filling pressures. *J. Am. Coll. Cardiol.* 1997; **30**: 1527–1533.

NAGUEH S.F., MIKATI I., KOPELEN H.A et al. Doppler estimation of left ventricular filling pressure in sinus tychycardia. A new application of tissue Doppler imaging. *Circulation* 1998; **98**: 1644–1650.

NISHIMURA R.A., TAJIK A.J. Evaluation of diastolic filling of left ventricule in health and disease: Doppler echocardiography is the clinician's Rosetta stone. *J. Am. Coll. Cardiol.* 1997; **30**: 8–18.

OH J.R., APPLETON C.P., HATLE L.K. et al. The non invasive assessment of left ventricular diastolic function with two dimensional and Doppler echocardiography. *J. Am. Soc. Echocardiogr.* 1997; **10**: 246–270.

OMMEN S.R., NISHIMURA R.A., APPLETON C.P. et al. Clinical utility of Doppler echocardiography and tissue Doppler imaging in the estimation of left ventricular filling pressures. *Circulation* 2000; **102**: 1788–1794.

OTTO C.M. *The Practice of Clinical Echocardiography.* Saunders, Philadelphia, 2002.

PALSKY D., LUTFALLA G. Méthodes d'évaluation de l'insuffisance cardiaque gauche par échocardiographie. *Réalités Cardiologiques* 1995; **86**: 16–32.

PANDIAN N., HSU T., SCHWARTZ S. et al. Multiplan transesophageal echocardiography. *Echocardiography* 1992; **9**: 649–666.

PATHE M. Analyse échographique de la diastole ventriculaire gauche. *Abs. Cardiol.* 2003; **383**: 20–23.

PERCHE H. Restriction-constriction. *Réalités Cardiologiques* 1994; **59**: 18–22.

PIERARD L. Insuffisance mitrale ischémique et insuffisance mitrale fonctionnelle. *La Lettre du Cardiologue* 2003; **370**: 11–12.

POP C., METZ D., TASSAN-MANGINA S. et al. Apport de l'échocardiographie Doppler sous dobutamine dans le rétrécissement aortique serré avec dysfonction ventriculaire gauche. *Arch. Mal. Cœur* 1999; **92**(11): 1487–1493.

PRUSZCZYC P., TORBICKI A., KUCH-WOCIAL A. et al. Transesophageal echocardiography for definitive diagnosis of haemodynamically significant pulmonary embolims. *Eur. Heart J.* 1995; **16**: 534–538.

QUERE J.P., LESBRE J.P. Diagnostic écho-Doppler des adiastolies. *Réalités Cardiologiques* 1997; **120**: 16–19.

RAFFOUL H. Critères échographiques pratiques de sévérité d'un rétrécissement aortique. *Cardiologie Pratique* 1997; **393**: 14–16.

RAFFOUL H. Diagnostic et évaluation d'une insuffisance ventriculaire gauche systolique. *Cardinale* 1997; **IX**(2): 31–39.

RAFFOUL H. Dilatation des cavités droites à l'échocardiographie. *Cardiologie Pratique* 1998; **438**: 11–14.

RAFFOUL H. Insuffisances aortiques; évaluation en écho-Doppler cardiaque et indications opératoires. *Cardiologie Pratique* 2000; **532**: 1–6.

RAFFOUL H., ABERGEL E. *Encyclopédie Pratique d'Echo-Doppler Cardiaque.* Squibb, Paris, 1992.

RAKOWSKI H., APPLETON C., CHAN K.L. et al. Canadian concensus recommendations for the measurement and reporting of diastolic dysfunction by echocardiography. *J. Am. Soc. Echocardiogr.* 1996; **9**: 736–760.

RASK L.P., KARP K.H., ERIKSSON N.P. Flow dependence of the aortic valve area in patients with aortic stenosis: assessment by application of continuity equation. *J. Am. Soc. Echocardiogr.* 1996; **9**(3): 295–299.

RODRIGUEZ L., ANCONINA F., FLACHSKAMPF F. et al. Impact of finite orifice on proximal flow convergence. Implications for Doppler quantification of valvular regurgitation. *Circulation Research* 1992; **70**: 923–930.

ROELANDT J. Three-dimensional echocardiography: new views from old windows. *Br. Heart J.* 1995; **74**: 4–6.

ROMAND S. *Échocardiographie du Chien et du Chat*. Thèse, École Nationale Vétérinaire de Lyon, 2002.

ROUDAUT R. Analyse morphologique de la valvule mitrale par échocardiographie. *La Lettre du Cardiologue* 1999; **311**: 27–31

ROUDAUT R. Échocardiographie tranœsophagienne et aorte thoracique douloureuse. *La Lettre du Cardiologue* 2000; **332**: 18–22.

ROUDAUT R. Les insuffisances valvulaires échocardiographiques sont-elles toujours pathologiques? *J. Faxe Cardiol.* March 1999.

ROUDAUT R. Place de l'échocardiographie dans la prise en charge de l'endocardite infectieuse. *Cardiologie Pratique* 1993; **246**: 1–3.

ROUDAUT R. Quelles sont les principales étiologies d'une obstruction dynamique du ventricule gauche? *Réalités Cardiologiques* 1997; **118**: 9–14.

ROUDAUT R. Signification du bourrelet septal sous-aortique. *Cardiologie Pratique* 1997; **407**: 16–18.

ROUDAUT R. Une pseudo-myocardiopathie hypertrophique. *La Lettre du Cardiologue* 1994; **221**: 14–15.

ROUDAUT R., DALLOCHIO M. L'hypertrophie septale asymétrique. *Cardiologie Pratique* 1990; **131**: 1–4.

ROUDAUT R., LABBE T., LEHERISSIER A., GOSSE P.H. Dissection aortique: diagnostic et surveillance par échocardiographie transthoracique et transœsophagienne. *Cardiologie Pratique* 1992; **223**: 7–9.

ROUDAUT R., LAFFORT P., LAFITTE S. et al. Place de l'échocardiographie dans le diagnostic des maladies acquises de l'aorte. *Arch. Mal. Coeur* 1997; **90**: 1687–1692.

ROUDAUT R., LATRABE V., MINIFIE C. et al. Hématome de la paroi thoracique: du diagnostic au traitement. *Arch. Mal. Cœur* 2000; **93**(4): 361–367.

ROUDAUT R., MARAZANOF M. Pièges échocardiographiques et dissection aortique. *Cardiologie Pratique* 1996; **369**: 1–7.

SCHEUBLE C. Péricardite constrictive. *Réalités Cardiologiques* 1995; **77**: 9–17.

SCHWAMMENTHAL E., POPESCU B.A., POPESCU A.C. et al. Non-invasive assessment of left ventricular end-diastolic pressure by the response of the transmitral A-wave velocity to a standardized Valsalva maneuver. *Am. J. Cardiol.* 2000; **86**: 169–174.

SCISLO P., KOCHANOWSKI J., KOSIOR D. Echocardiography in non-invasive diagnosis in left ventricular heart failure. *Terapia (Kardiologia)* 2003; **9**(142): 12–15.

SLAMA M.A., JOBIC Y. Les myocardiopathies hypertrophiques: classification et investigation par écho-Doppler. *Cardioscopies* 1996; **42**: 220–224.

SOHN D.W., CHAI I.H., LEE D.J. et al. Assessment of mitral annulus velocity by Doppler tissue imaging in the evaluation of left ventricular diastolic function. *J. Am. Coll. Cardiol.* 1997; **30**: 474–480.

SOHN D.W., SONG J.M., ZO J.H. et al. Mitral annulus velocity in the evaluation of left ventricular diastolic function in atrial fibrillation. *J. Am. Soc. Echocardiogr.* 1999; **12**: 927–931.

TOUCHE T. L'insuffisance mitrale diastolique. *Réalités Cardiologiques* 1994; **65**: 13–16.

TRIBOUILLOY C. *Échocardiographie Transœsophagienne.* Médecine-Sciences Flammarion, Paris, 1994.

TRIBOUILLOY C. Qu'est ce que la PISA. *Arch. Mal. Coeur Pratique* 1996; **28**: 16–18.

TRIBOUILLOY C., GOISSEN T. Quantification des régurgitations valvulaires par la méthode de convergence. *Cardiologie Pratique* 2002; **619**: 12–14.

TRIBOUILLOY C., LESBRE J.P. *Échocardiographie des Cardiopathies Valvulaires Acquises.* Médecine-Sciences Flammarion, Paris, 1993.

TRIBOUILLOY C., MIRODE A., LESBRE J.P. Comment apprécier la sévérité d'une insuffisance mitrale en écho-Doppler? *Cardinale* 1996, **VIII**(5): 35–39.

TRIBOUILLOY C., MIRODE A., LESBRE J.P. Échographie transœsophagienne et quantification des insuffisances mitrales. *Réalités Cardiologiques* 1997; **113**: 11–13.

TRIBOUILLOY C., MIRODE A., LESBRE J.P. Quantification d'une insuffisance mitrale par écho-Doppler transthoracique. *Réalités Cardiologiques* 1997; **113**: 5–10.

TRIBOUILLOY C., MIRODE A., ROUDAUT R., LESBRE J.P. ETO et pathologie aortique. *Arch. Mal. Cœur Prat.* 1966; **24**: 18–21.

TRIBOUILLOY C., PELTIER M. Quantification des insuffisances mitrales par l'étude de la zone de convergence intra-ventriculaire gauche. *Réalités Cardiologiques* 1993; **49**: 32–40.

TRIBOUILLOY C., QUERE J.P., LESBRE J.P. Enregistrement du flux veineux pulmonaire par échocardiographie doppler: aspects normaux et pathologiques. *Arch. Mal. Coeur* 1995; **88**: 1335–1344.

TSANG T.S., OH J.K., SEWARD J.R. Diagnosis and management of cardiac tamponade in the era of echocardiography. *Clin. Cardiol.* 1999; **22**: 446–452.

VACHERON A. Prolapsus valvulaire mitral. Qu'en est-il en l'an 2000? *Cardiologie Pratique* 2000; **525**: 9–12.

VAHANIAN A. et al. Intégrale: rétrécissement aortique calcifié. *Cardiologie* 2000; **546**.

VEYRAT C., PELLERIN D., LARRAZE F. Imagerie Doppler tissulaire du myocarde: passé, présent et avenir. *Arch. Mal. Coeur* 1997; **90**(10): 1391–1401.

XIE G.Y., BERK M.R., SMITH M.D. et al. Relation of Doppler transmitral flow patterns to functional status in congestive heart failure. *Am. Heart J.* 1996; **131**: 766–771.

Index

S

SAM *see* systolic anterior motion
sampling volume 15
sector field, angle 12–13
septal kinking 36, 102–3, 150
septal rim 36, 102, 105, 109, 116, 118,
    150
shadow cone 6
shortening fraction (SF) 157–9
sinus tachycardia 32
sinus of Valsalva 69, 73
    aneurysm 218
spectral Doppler, pitfalls 14–15
spectrum speed 15
spontaneous contrast 152, 154, 155
stenotic flow 42–6
stenotic jet, incomplete recording 26
strands, fibrin 69, 150
stress/exercise echocardiography 47,
    115, 116, 122, 207
stretching phenomenon 122
stunning phenomenon 124
subaortic diameter 36–9, 162, 164
subaortic flows 39–42
subhepatic venous flow (SHVF) 198
    systolic fraction 198–9
surface shortening fraction (SSF)
    184–5
swinging heart 133–4
systolic anterior motion (SAM) 112,
    113, 114, 117
    false 113, 133
systolic function
    of left ventricle 157–65
    of right ventricle 184–5

T

Teicholz formula 159, 160
tendons, false 99–100, 150
Theile sinus 73, 208, 211
three-dimensional echocardiography
    162
thrombus 126, 152, 153, 208, 215, 220
    in left atrial appendage 149
time gain compensation (TGC) 13
trabeculations, coarse 150
transoesophageal echocardiography
    (TEE) 21, 24, 73, 207

trans-stenotic pressure gradient 25–7
transthoracic echocardiography (TTE)
    24
tricuspid flow 187–8
tricuspid regurgitation (TR) 44,
    193–200
    laminar 199
    physiological 53
    trivial 199
tricuspid stenosis 202
turbulence 16, 88
two-dimensional echocardiography
    54–64

U

ultrasonic waves, physical properties 3

V

Valsalva manoeuvre 115, 180, 181,
    197
valve mobility 23
valvular leaks 49–90
    aetiology 53–73
    Doppler analysis 75–90
    haemodynamic consequences 74–5
    physiological vs pathological 51–3
    small, ultrasound artefacts vs 50–1,
        52
valvular regurgitation 74
    see also aortic regurgitation; mitral
        regurgitation
valvular stenoses 21–49
    see also aortic stenosis; mitral
        stenosis
vegetations 65–70, 152
    non-infective 68
    obstructive 69–70
velocity–time integral (VTI) 36, 38,
    42, 43, 80, 162
vena contracta 40, 75, 78–9, 91
ventricular dilatation 141–3
ventricular segments 125

W

wall hypertrophy 95, 110–12, 179
    compensatory 125
    see also left ventricular hypertrophy
Wolf–Parkinson–White syndrome 159